THE DIET-WHISPERER

Dr Paul Barrington Chell
Dr Monique Hope-Ross

Copyright © 2020 MediaMedica Ltd

First published in Great Britain in 2020

www.diet-whisperer.com

The moral right of MediaMedica Ltd to be identified as the author of this work has been asserted in accordance with the Copyright, Designs and Patents Act 1988.

A CIP catalog record for this book is available from the British Library.

ISBN 979-8-66789-218-2

Every effort has been made to fulfill copyright requirements with regard to reproducing copyright material. The author and publisher will be glad to rectify any omissions at the earliest opportunity.

The book is intended to provide helpful information related to health issues. Every effort has been made to ensure that the information in this book is accurate. The author and publisher assume no responsibility for errors, inaccuracies, omissions or inconsistencies herein.

This book is not intended to prevent, diagnose, treat or cure any condition or disease. Please consult with your health care specialist regarding the suggestions and recommendations made in this book. The author and publisher are not responsible for any damages or negative consequences to any person reading or following the information in this book. References are provided for information and do not constitute endorsement of any websites or sources. The use of this book implies your acceptance of this disclaimer.

Published by Amazon

To our mothers, Maureen and Claire and our late fathers, Derick and Daniel

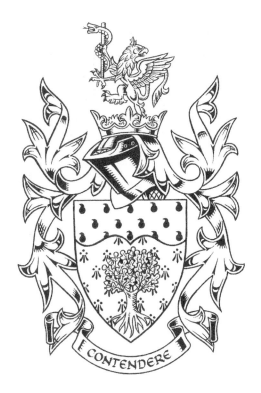

CONTENTS

"Take back control. See instant results. Become the diet-whisperer for you and your loved ones."

PBC & MHR; Whisperer HQ

PART ONE: THE ROAD TO OBESITY

PART TWO: THE ROAD TO PERMANENT WEIGHT LOSS

ABOUT THE AUTHORS

Dr Paul Barrington Chell MB ChB FRCOphth DO (RCSI)

Dr Monique Hope-Ross MB ChB BAO FRCP FRCS FRCOphth DO

Paul and Monique went to medical school in Birmingham UK and University College Dublin respectively. Following their residencies and early careers in general medicine and surgery, both specialized in Ophthalmic Surgery, where they met as junior doctors. They were married in 1995. They held fellowships at Moorfields Eye Hospital, London and Manhattan Eye and Ear Hospital, New York. Paul was appointed consultant ophthalmic surgeon to Worcester Eye Infirmary in 1996, where the team gained national recognition as a "Beacon Site" for excellence in cataract surgery in 2000. He specialized in corneal transplant surgery, and for many years performed all transplant surgery for the whole of Worcestershire and surrounding counties. Monique was appointed to the Birmingham and Midland Eye Hospital in 1993, where she also held the post of honorary senior lecturer at the university of Birmingham, UK. She specialized in diseases of the retina. Between them they spent 20 years as head of departments. They both retired from ophthalmic surgery in 2016, to pursue their desire to work in the field of preventative nutrition, recognizing the severity of the obesity pandemic.

They have five university degrees, are diplomats of the Royal College of Surgeons of England and Ireland and are Fellows of four Royal Medical Colleges in the United Kingdom.

They have each delivered over 100 invited scientific lectures and have written many book chapters. They have over 100 scientific publications, abstracts and communications to their names. They have both been scientific reviewers for international scientific journals. For the past 10 years they have delivered invited lectures on nutrition, health and wellness.

Paul and Monique have been Trustees to many charities and were elected Presidents of five national and international learned medical societies.

Outside of work they are both keen skiers. They started doing triathlons in their fifties. Paul did his first Olympic distance triathlon in 2016, at the age of 55, and Monique her first Ironman 140.6 in 2019 at the age of 59.

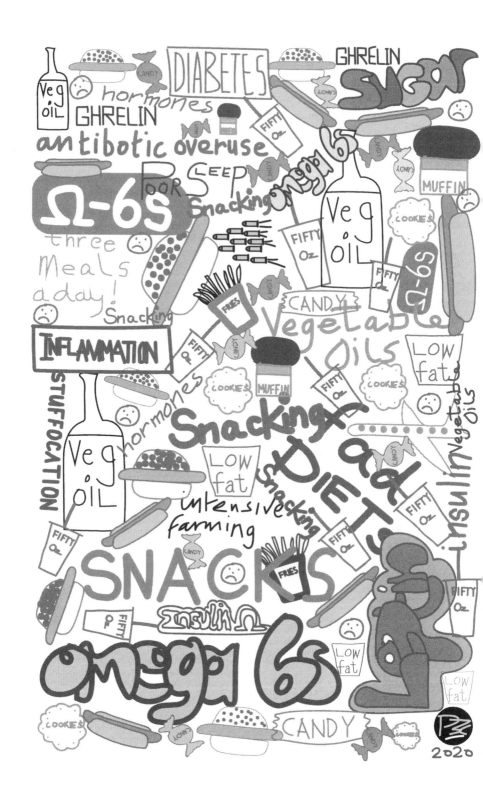

PART ONE

THE ROAD TO OBESITY

CHAPTER 1

ABOUT THIS BOOK

"Salad. I can't bear salad. It grows while you're eating it you know."

Alan Ayckbourn

WHO IS THE BOOK DESIGNED FOR?

Firstly, a very big welcome to the diet-whisperer family. Monique and I are both doctors and wrote this book for all like-minded individuals; anyone wanting to lose weight and keep it off. And we'll certainly show you how to do that. But it's very much more than just weight; it's about putting you in control and helping you improve your mental and physical health. And, helping people to understand the way food influences chronic inflammatory diseases; leaving people in pain and disabled for decades. We know from science that diets work for a while, but eventually fail. The whisperer plan is not a diet. It is a journey where you learn a lifestyle that you can adopt forever and love it. On the journey you will learn facts that will shatter long-held beliefs and preconceptions. The whole idea of the whisperer plan is to put you firmly back in control of your own body. You will choose your target weight and achieve your goals. You will learn the foods that make you ill. You will see immediate results from your actions, as you join us on this exciting journey.

It is a book for men and women, young or old. Whilst not a medical textbook, we hope doctors and medical students will enjoy it, and learn from it too. We have pitched it at all people who are inquisitive to know more about the relationship between obesity, illness, food and our fat storage hormones. Our readers share a common goal; they know that our current nutrition is causing us obesity, great harm and illness. And they feel out of control and unable to get help. We will show you how and why, and the ways to

3

correct those wayward hormones. And you will see that by us all acting in harmony, how we will benefit our societies too.

HOW TO USE THIS BOOK

The first half of the book is "the road to obesity" and the second half "the road to permanent weight loss". If you ask me which is more important, I'm bound to say both. But I want to emphasize how important the first half is, because it gets you more than halfway to the solution. In other words, when you know what causes obesity, and most people don't, you have a great deal of empowerment. Whilst stating the obvious, the order of the chapters is carefully chosen so you will learn by gently, layering up your knowledge as you go. I can promise you some Eureka moments in every chapter, and where you least expect them. We finish each chapter with a summary, chapter whisperings, and there is a glossary to help you at the back of the book.

You do not need to have any medical or scientific knowledge to read this book; just a desire to be leaner, healthier and live longer. It sounds obvious, but we wanted to start with this before you go diving into the whisperer plans. We understand that you are mad keen to lose 44 pounds (c. 20 kg) in 20 weeks. But it is important to go steadily through this book, chapter by chapter, building your knowledge, for a completely different outlook on life. The new you. And even better, it will put you back in control of your body and in a position to help your loved ones too.

Monique has written the chapters on Wheat and Gluten, The Microbiome and Wellness. I'm afraid you'll have to put up with me for rest. For the record, this has been a joint project for the last ten years. Start to finish, and we've loved every minute of the journey and have both worked hard to make this project work for you. When you regain complete 100% control over your own body weight, join us on the website and let us know how you're doing. Make us happy at whisperer HQ.

METABOLIC SYNDROME AND DIABETES

If you have type 2 diabetes and would like to give yourself a chance of reversing it. Or if you have pre-diabetes, or metabolic syndrome, this can be of the utmost, life changing importance to you. Invest your time in learning about food, your fat storage hormones and how they interact. Don't worry about any of these terms for now, they will all become second nature by the end. You will need your physician on board to adjust your medications, as you lose weight rapidly. There is no single cure, pill or magic bullet. But, when you finish the book, you will understand enough to free yourself from the control of the fad diet companies, and the poisonous food sellers. You will be in control of your own destiny. You will be able to choose your weight and most importantly control it long-term. On our website there are lots of resources to help improve your health. We encourage you to do the fun quiz before and after reading the book. Its confidential and will show you how much your knowledge has changed.

When you register you will be eligible for our blogs and health bulletins on the latest science and medical issues of the day. If like us you've failed so many times with diets, it's time you became your own diet-whisperer and take control over your hormones, nutrition and weight. Learn to help yourself and the loves one's around you. That's the essence of what we're about. Learning then spreading the word; helping others and improving your karma.

Thanks for getting this far. We hope you enjoy the journey. Welcome to the whisperer family.

Paul and Monique

Dr Paul Barrington Chell and Dr Monique Hope-Ross
Medical Directors
The diet-whisperer.

CHAPTER 2

INTRODUCTION

"If you think that low-fat diets, and low-fat yogurt, will help you lose weight, you should definitely read on."

PBC & MHR; Whisperer HQ

TWO SURGEONS

It was Friday evening and Monique and I were heading home. As usual our Friday clinics had run over, with many patients wanting to be seen before the weekend. In medicine, Friday afternoons and Monday mornings are always busiest. Our routine was to telephone each other at halfway on our 40-mile commute. For Monique this was when she passed the Belfry, home to the Brabazon golf course and four Ryder cups. Halfway for me was less salubrious, simply where I left the Northbound M5 motorway for the Eastbound M42. I have a tendency to swear at the BBC radio news, so at the end of a long week, had turned the radio off; I needed some silence. Even so, I was pleased to see Monique's name come up on the screen, and we chatted for ten minutes as usual. We never chatted for too long, respecting each other's need for peace. A kind of buffer between the stress of the day job and the peace of our beautiful Warwickshire farm. On summer evenings we would pass through Henley-in-Arden, a medieval town with a high street rich in architecture, history and our friends sitting outside the bars enjoying the sunshine. The high street runs north to south, so the bars are on the left facing the evening sun. Always a joyous scene of laughter and conviviality; a source of vicarious pleasure and a little envy. This time I passed through ahead of Monique. We had a rule that "first home" fed the dogs and would be there to give a special warm welcome to "second home". Kay, our thoughtful housekeeper and friend, ensured our home was beautiful and arranged flowers in the kitchen. In the summer, I would take the dogs out for a walk around our beautiful farm; in the middle of nowhere and with eye watering views. I would sit high up on a natural bank, looking down onto the long driveway where the dogs sat in anticipation and could recognize the sound of Monique's car as she approached the gates. The creak from the gates and dogs became trembling wrecks of anticipation. Dogs give love to their family, but only have one master, and that was Monique. I was never too sure where I fell in the pecking order!

As Monique arrived, I reflected on our earlier conversation. I could always tell when she had something on her mind. The car stopped and I released the dogs. As usual, they raced to greet her. Three sentient beings and a moment of intemperate pleasure. The two dogs would then race each other around the croquet lawn showing off to impress, as us boys do. We went inside for supper and as we chatted, I opened a bottle of 1986 Palmer. Monique told me that Jane, a patient in her twenties and whom we had shared, was now totally blind. The result of diabetes and its effect on the eye. My earlier question answered.

We were always affected, deeply and personally by poor outcomes in our patients. This was a weakness, not a strength. For years, we had witnessed so many of our patients on a pathway to personal Armageddon; poor nutrition, obesity, insulin resistance, metabolic syndrome, diabetes and blindness. And it wasn't just us. In cardiology, it was the same pathway, ending in heart attacks and strokes, in vascular surgery ending in amputations and in nephrology ending in kidney failure. Every specialty was touched by this epidemic. All because of the way that we humans had come to interact with our planet; with nature and in particular our nutrition. Patients with blood pressure are given pills, yet we know they get better outcomes from a daily 30-minute walk.[1,2] We had started seeing this as a nonsense. In eye surgery, treatment of advanced diabetic eye disease involves laser destruction of the peripheral retina, to save the central sight; such a painful and preventable waste of life and resources.

Monique and I had reached the top of our profession as eye surgeons. We had maintained our deep interests in medicine, nutrition and biochemistry. For ten years we had been researching nutrition for our patients, with a particular emphasis on obesity reduction and wellness. We had lectured at home and abroad to GPs, surgeons, optometrists, hospital staff, allied professionals and the public about nutritional causes of long-term health problems.

That night at the supper table, the conversation was different. Fueled by the red truth syrup, we decided to go the whole hog and retire from the day job. Stop the surgical careers completely. We would work full time on the prevention of long-term disease. We would give people a different option of how they interacted with their planet, with a particular emphasis on nutrition. In the modern globally connected village, we could reach far more people and get to them early. We were to go from being treatment doctors to prevention doctors. This was a big decision, and in our house a big decision goes on the six-week board. The cork from that wine went onto the six-week board too; both of which exist to this day. The irony of the cork being 1986, the year I qualified as a doctor. Six weeks later we became prevention doctors.

THE CHALLENGE

The challenge was simple; we have an obesity epidemic and diets don't work. To be truthful, they all work for a while, then the pounds all come back on. And people pay out good money for this predictable cycle of success followed by failure. Yes, at six-months the weight is down, with reduced cardiovascular risks of heart attacks and strokes. But the scientific evidence tells us at twelve months, the weight comes back and the risks return.[1] Worse still, every time your diet fails, you enter the yo-yo diet phenomenon. You lose not only fat, but also muscle. When the weight returns, you replace it with fat. Yo-yo dieting accelerates the rate of muscle loss from the body at a rate that resembles the seriously ill. It makes us get weaker as we get older. Repeated dieting is bad for us all and science tells us that the answer does not lie here.

THE SEARCH

Perhaps if we looked at how societies had changed over the last fifty years, would we find the correlation or causation there? And over time we certainly did. Changes in religious beliefs, smoking habits, divorce rates, single parenting and moving away from hometowns for work. They were all implicated. It was hard to imagine that seemingly unrelated things would contribute too; like cesarean sections and the widespread use of antibiotics in humans and in farming, but they did! And what about the Blue Zones in the world, where people not only enjoy a longer lifespan, but also have a longer healthspan, free from illness, pills and doctors. I use the word "enjoy" judiciously. Monique and I had concluded a long time ago that pills are bad. In our research we found both correlations and causations, that related to so many aspects of modern life.

On this voyage of discovery, we learned that only a fool would think obesity had one cause and that the cure to obesity would be one single answer. Or, what works for one person would work equally well for another. We also learned there is most definitely an answer to both personal and societal obesity. Individuals and society have changed. Changes that are likely irreversible, in the main. So, if we cannot un-change society, we need a solution that fits today's lifestyles, and preferably with some built in future proofing.

COMBINATION THERAPY

In our early years, Monique and I both worked in cancer therapy. So often, we waited with great expectancy for the next big breakthrough; the monoclonal antibody treatments and immunotherapy that have since revolutionized cancer care. But we remember those old cancer research units, where we spent our evenings mixing up the next day's chemotherapy. And where almost none of the treatments were truly novel, but rather new combinations of old treatments. Much like the early days of HIV. Combination treatments, that hit the sweet spot; combination treatments where the sum of the parts was greater than the whole. Monique and I began to realize that by combining traditional treatments with our modern understanding of hormones, we could provide a long-lasting solution to weight control. And most importantly, it wouldn't require the fads, diet shakes and sleight of hand used by diet company fraudsters. People would have the tools to put them back in charge of their own bodies, and they could then determine their own weight and health.

FAT ADAPTATION

There were several areas of interest that combined to form the whole. We had been working with athletes on nutrition, hydration and electrolyte balance. We had for many years been progressively, and somewhat intermittently, reducing refined carbohydrates in our own diet. And we knew the beneficial effects of omega-3 fats on life expectancy. Monique had lectured on the gut microbiome and bringing all of these things together, it seemed that the sum of the parts may exceed the whole. But the thing is, even applying these principles to ourselves, we had the same outcome. Weight off for a while, then it all came back again, much to our frustration. We will cover why this happens in later chapters. We had many of the right factors but not all of them.

Latterly, we had been working on fat adaptation for endurance sports, like triathlon. Many athletes were, like the rest of society, in a twentieth-century sort of way, completely attuned to pre-loading, fueling and recovering on carbohydrates. Science said that carbohydrate was the best fuel for sport including endurance. Like the others, we had also been fueling our sports activity on carbohydrates.

Like a hybrid car that runs on gas (petrol) or electricity, we are too a duel fuel system. Our ancestors ran almost exclusively on fats, and we run almost exclusively on carbs. The thing is that our modern bodies have been tuned to only burn carbs. Every meal, snack and drink has taught our bodies to be tuned to burning carbohydrates. This happens not through the consumption of nutritious vegetables rich in fiber, but flour-based and sugar-based refined carbohydrate food and drinks. This is why we need fat adaption, to allow us to burn fat once again. You will learn to control the hormones that prevent fat burning in the 21st century. Just think about yesterday's meals. Worse still, we often don't know what types of food were in the meal we ate.

Imagine filling up a car and not caring or knowing what fuel you put in; gas (petrol) or diesel, who cares! That would hold up as reasonable evidence for insanity. Yet with food, not knowing what basic nutrients we're eating is normal. So, the first part of the diet-whisperer plan, is to empower you with the simple knowledge of our basic foodstuffs, carbohydrates, fats and proteins. You will learn some shocking things along the way.

The diet-whisperer is about empowering you with knowledge to put you back in control. For decades in endurance sport, it has been known that we can re-tune our bodies to burn fat. This process is called fat adaptation. And when endurance athletes fat adapt, they can go longer and harder than science thought possible. Most importantly, if we could teach non-athletes fat adaptation, they could happily burn fat all day long; at work, at play or vegging in the evening watching TV. And here is the logic. If fat adapted athletes can learn to run fifty-mile ultramarathons on their endless stores of body fat, why can't we fat adapt everyone. Was this even possible? And how successfully would it crossover into more sedentary lifestyles?

THE CLOCK: FASTSPAN ® AND EATSPAN ®

The more we worked on foods for fat adaptation, the more we combined it with altered mealtimes. This was to stimulate new fat burning pathways in the body. This is as old as the hills and can be traced back to Greek philosophers. The time period between the last morsel to cross your lips at night and the first one in the morning gives us the name of the first meal of the day; breakfast, or break-the-fast! It is of fundamental importance as you will learn, and we call this the FastSpan.

There are two other vitally important aspects to food and timing. Firstly, the time period from your first food of the day to the last which we call the EatSpan. And the second is the number of meals taken within the EatSpan. At the whisperer, there is no such thing as a snack; we call all snacks a meal and you should too from now onward. The importance of this will become crystal clear as your journey unwinds.

AUTOPHAGY

It is extraordinary that most of the work on anti-aging has a common theme, autophagy. Pronounced 'ort-off-a-gee'. It means the hoovering up of the aging components within our cells, by round fatty globules called lysosomes. To your cell it's like changing the old oil and replacing worn engine parts in the car. It's a process of renewal. Autophagy slows down with aging and bits of large molecules and mitochondria, start to lie around in our cells, rather than getting vacuumed up. A bit like my study writing this book with piles of paper everywhere. When we look at the aging skin, the fibroblast cells that keep our skin smooth and elastic, are getting stuffed up with their own products of intracellular life. In aging, the renewal and repair processes that keep these cells fit and healthy are failing. The two most powerful tools to increase autophagy are fasting and exercise.

THE SOLUTION

So, like our old oncology jobs, we might be able to reverse-engineer and combine these factors into a twenty-first century package that works. It must be flexible enough to respect the emotional, physiological and psychological differences between us. It must be flexible enough to allow us to err and regain control quickly. Like most men, I tend to go dietary off-piste more than Monique, who is better disciplined. Over the years as Monique and I worked on this nutrition plan, it became obvious there was always one common factor. One glue that created success, as well as failure. One factor that controlled everything including us. Our hormones; specifically, our nutritional hormones. And that is how the diet-whisperer was born.

THE DIET-WHISPERER PLAN

We started with a 12-week program targeting 26 pounds (12 kg or 1.88 stone) of weight loss; which was ambitious but safe. There is a basic and powerful transition of three transitional blocks, each lasting 4 weeks;

1. The 1st is to achieve a state of fat adaption through dietary manipulation

2. The 2nd is to enhance fat burning pathways by manipulating EatSpan and FastSpan

3. The 3rd is to combine 1 and 2 further to reach your stated target, with you now in control of your fat storage hormones. This section can be lengthened until target weight is achieved. Then we will be able to add in some treat foods as and when you wish to.

No magic, just methods based on science, putting you in the driving seat of your own destiny. Monique and I realized that once you learned the basic rules, you could then control your own hormones. When you control your hormones, you control your weight. You can then decide your weight and you can get there. And once you get there, you can stay there. You are then free; free from diet foods, diet clubs and all that nonsense and madness.

You do not need to be a doctor to understand this book. We promise you a journey of discovery. When you have completed the book, you will be able to choose your weight, achieve your weight and maintain your weight. And Monique and I shall be delighted with your new ability to control your weight, shape and wellness. You will feel great and be able to control your fat storage hormones; you will be a diet-whisperer.

MY PERSONAL EXPERIENCE WITH THE DIET-WHISPERER PROGRAM

I had been trying for years trying to trim down. As with all dieters I had lost weight, then put it back on, lost weight, put it back on, and followed the classical yo-yo diet pattern. At 58 years old and 6-feet-tall (180 cm), I weighed in at 213 pounds (96.6 kg or 15 stone).

Monique and I modified the whisperer plan for me, taking it out to twenty weeks rather than twelve, which is easy to do once the first 2 transitions are complete. I wanted to lose 44 pounds (20 kg or 3 stone) in 20 weeks. Not only did I achieve this, but my weight is now stable at 170 pounds (77 Kg or 12.1 stone). That was over one year ago.

If I put a few pounds on, I can lose them in the same week. And we'll show you how to do that. I am the same weight one year later. My abdominal girth went down from 42 inches to 30 inches (105 cm to 75 cm), reduced by one foot! My blood pressure came down, to a systolic of under 110 mmHg. I feel physically and mentally stronger than I have for years. I take no tablets and have a normal cholesterol profile. I still enjoy, gin, beer and wine! I eat normal foods at the right times and respect my EatSpan and FastSpan. I alternate my normal foods with treats and a ketogenic diet. Somedays vegetarian, somedays not, creating a balance that I'm happy with.

In the 20 weeks and 44 pounds weight loss period, I did zero exercise. That's right; zero exercise, not even a long walk. I did this to show my fellow diet-whisperers that to get thin, you need to control your hormones; no exercise required. The gym comes later, and you will learn the merits of this. We can cite so many more diet-whisperers, that have very similar stories to mine. We had a call from a man's wife last week, telling us that "for the first time in his adult life his weight is in the normal range". What pleasure we got from that! Just like watching our patients recovering from eye surgery; there is no greater joy than helping others. And karma is great for wellness.

In the following chapters, we will show you how to lose weight by controlling your hormones. But, the first thing you must know is that if you shout at your hormones, they'll beat you. Their powers are so strong, they will either destroy you, or make you thrive. Learn to whisper to them, and you'll learn to harness their power; power that has meant your ancestors have survived since man first stood upright. You will learn to control your hormones and hence your weight and shape. You will have learned the secret to a long and healthy life. Welcome new whisperer.

THE PHILOSOPHY OF THE DIET-WHISPERER

This is quite simple. There is a mountain of information out there today. But because of its medical nature, it doesn't pass easily to people of a non-scientific background. It's easy to lose the simple messages with medical jargon. This book is here to help you to understand what you need to understand to be able to access that information. Monique and I have spent our whole working lives teaching peers and juniors and explaining complicated concepts to our patients. We regarded this as a central part of what we do. When you finish the book, you will have developed the skills needed to decide your weight, get there and stay there. We won't tell you what to eat at every hour of every day, or sell you ridiculous powdered drinks, or even make you eat horrid low-calorie foods. No, you will be able to go to the market, buy fresh food and know what you want to eat, and when you want to eat it. You are the only person that knows which food you like, and so as a principle it should be you that decides. You will learn to get back on track if you wander, and you will wander, if you're anything like me! You will be able to enjoy a drink and a meal with friends; you will value that time and the joy of such occasions without guilt. Your food plan must not be at the expense of a robust and healthy social life.

With our help, you will build a framework of nutrition; specifically, for you. You will then be able to furnish that framework and build your own healthy food plan. You may supplement with paleo, keto or vegan. Names don't matter. It is the principles of "what food", and "when food", that are the critical things to know. The most important thing is you understand what it is you're trying to achieve. Only then will you be on your new path for life, you will have joined the rest of us that can whisper to our hormones. Welcome to the whisperer family.

CHAPTER WHISPERINGS

- Obesity leads to every department in the hospital
- Science tells us that diets don't work; they work for a while then fail
- Changes in lifestyle over 50 years have impacted on our weight
- Combination therapies, are more powerful than the sum of the parts for weight control
- Fat adaptation, learning to live off our fat is possible for athletes and sedentary adults
- EatSpan and FastSpan are critical to weight control

- Reduced autophagy leads to aging; the whisperer plan increases autophagy
- The important common factor to all weight gain and weight loss is our hormones

My personal experience with the diet-whisperer program was very successful, meeting both my short-term and long-term goals.

Last reminder; please have some fun and do the quiz on the website before you get into the book, so you can monitor how much you've learned by doing it again at the end; it's a bit of fun!

Disclaimer

The Diet-Whisperer represents our views and experiences and under no circumstance does it constitute medical advice. It was a movement born after leaving clinical medicine and has no connection whatsoever with the people or places we worked in. Although we are both medical doctors, we advise you see your doctor before embarking on any advice in this book. And, encourage your doctors to read it too! This plan is not suitable for children. By working with your physician and the lessons in this book, there is a possibility you can reverse type 2 diabetes. If you have diabetes, take advice from your physician about hypoglycemia and if you're on antihypertensive treatment about low blood pressure too. Your physician may have to supervise withdrawal of your medications to prevent excessive lowering of your blood pressure and or blood glucose. If you have any medical condition, or psychological eating problems, you should not implement this, or any other nutrition plan without discussing it with your doctor first. If your doctor refuses to help, no problem, you need a new doctor; move on. Assumptions are made in discussing hormones and physiology, that changes and causes are not from underlying health conditions. We assume good health as the baseline for discussions.

CHAPTER 3

THE OBESITY PANDEMIC

"Thou seest I have more flesh than another man, and therefore more frailty."
William Shakespeare, Henry IV.

INTRODUCTION

Obesity is not caused by over-eating and lying around. Obese people are not lazy people and only lazy thinkers believe that. Like most long-term conditions, obesity's origins lie in a complex mixture of factors; a veritable minestrone soup. With certainty, it is a mixture of nature and nurture. Nature is our genes which are responsible for around 70% of obesity. Nurture is responsible for the rest.

We cannot alter our genes, but the nurture part we can. Nurture means environment, which means everything that is not genetic. It means your place and date of birth, your school, your job, where you live, pollution, pesticides, fertilizers, noise, stress, wealth, education, your partner, your country, your habits, exercise and fitness, what time you go to bed and rise, your food, how many times a day you eat, snacking, alcohol, smoking, drugs, soft drink habits, the weather, the altitude of your home, the terrain you live around, working shifts, travel, methods of travel, occupation, your hobbies, your pets, your neighbors, your family, your social group or tribe, the method of delivery when you were born and the environmental factors your mother was exposed to whilst carrying you, including her diet. So, in obesity, nature is your genes, and nurture is everything else in your life.

THE NOT-SO-FUN NUMBERS

Financially, we are drowning in obesity debt. In the USA, obesity alone is costing $150 Billion a year. Interestingly, that money equates to the entire cost of the UK's National Health Service, treating 67 million people free at the point of service for one full year. Taking the last ten years growth in health spend versus GDP and modeling it forwards, the US health budget will reach 50% of GDP by 2035. The US health budget will surpass GDP in 2047. In very simple terms, if America doesn't deal with the obesity epidemic, the US will go bust in less than 30 years. Australia will be bust by 2066 and the UK in 2086. Not only is obesity killing us individually, but it's going to bankrupt our great nations.

We measure obesity in individuals by body mass index (BMI). It is a calculation based on height and weight. It allows us to compare country to country quite well. It is less good for individuals because of differences in build types. You can calculate your own BMI on our website. Underweight is below 18.5, normal is 18.5 to 24.9, overweight is 25.0 to 29.9 and obese is over 30.0. So, in comparing countries we look at two figures. The first is the percentage of the population with a BMI >30, and the second is the average BMI for that country amongst all its people.

You may be surprised to read that it is not the USA and UK leading the global obesity stakes, and we are ranked 12th and 36th respectively. That honor goes to Polynesian and Caribbean countries, closely followed by the Gulf states and led by Kuwait.[3] Oil rich countries are piling on the pounds in the Middle East, and importantly as Islamic Kingdoms they are booze free. In 2020, more than 2.1 billion of our fellow humans are obese globally; 30% of the world's population.

WHO reports show globally 3 million deaths each year can be attributed to obesity and over 41 million preschool children are obese and will die prematurely. In American Samoa, a fantastical 74.6 % of the population are obese, and the population has an average BMI of 34.9. As comparators, the USA has a 36.2% obesity rate, with the population average BMI 28.8; that is a staggering 119 million obese people. In the UK, the figures are 27.8% obese, with an average Brit's BMI being 27.3. Again, that equates to 19

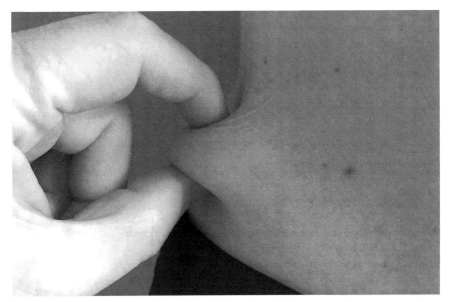

Figure 2.1. Pinching an inch of subcutaneous fat.

million people with a BMI over 30. And whilst only 6.2% of Chinese are obese with a good average BMI of 23.9, their population size means that they have a staggering 89 million obese people with BMI's over 30. At the bottom of the list is Vietnam, with only 2.1% obese and the country's average BMI is 21.6.

It's very important to define the two major types of fat. Firstly, the pinch an inch type, examples being on your arms, legs or belly (figure 2.1). This is called subcutaneous fat, our wobbly bits. Secondly, the really dangerous fat lies inside the belly and is known as visceral fat. Visceral fat is hormonally active and is now regarded as an organ in its own right. You cannot feel your visceral fat because it is deep inside. You will only notice its size as it pushes out your waistline and belt size. This is the killer fat, that leads to metabolic syndrome and the diseases discussed below.

Let's continue with the numbers. The obesity epidemic is the cause of "Peak Age". For those readers not familiar with this term, I have borrowed it from the oil exploration and production industry, where "peak oil" represents that time when a tipping point in a well's production is reached and oil output starts to decrease from that moment forwards. I have been sifting through the annual accounts of some of the world's biggest Life Assurance Companies, and they, or rather their very smart actuaries, seem to agree with me; that Peak Age is upon us. In other words, for the first time in 100 years, the rise in life expectancy is slowing. The "death contingencies" of Life Assurance Companies are being reduced. These are financial provisions, put to one side to cope with the pension demands of increasing life expectancy. One such company, Legal and General listed on the FTSE 100, reduced death contingencies by $160 and $300 million in 2017 and 2018 respectively.[4] And, they believe this so strongly, they're going around buying up the pension liabilities of many large corporations. My words not theirs, but still strong stuff.

There is some great news. Firstly, we can now diagnose visceral fat and metabolic syndrome early, and independent of your size. Secondly, when we do, we can turn it around. And thirdly you get to feel a whole bunch better straight way. The whisperer plan will put you back in control.

OBESITY, VISCERAL FAT AND METABOLIC SYNDROME: THE CONSEQUENCES

Metabolic syndrome is a condition that occurs silently without symptoms. It is a cluster of conditions; visceral fat, high blood pressure (hypertension) and high blood sugar (glucose), high triglycerides and high bad cholesterol (LDL). If you are obese you have an 80% chance of visceral fat and metabolic syndrome. When visceral fat and metabolic syndrome occur, the next stops on the bus route are diabetes type 2, cardiovascular disease and premature death. Sorry, blunt but true. Some of the commonest associated medical conditions are listed below.[5,6]

- Cancer: obesity is proven to be the biggest cause of cancer, after smoking

- Holy Trinity: obesity, smoking and lack of exercise leads to morbidity and death at a very early age

- Silent death: obesity doesn't hurt. It causes few symptoms for many years, then health fails suddenly, leading to long-term illness and early death

- Sleep: sleep is the biggest healer in our day, relieving stresses and helping to repair our bodies and repair the earliest cellular changes of many types of cancer. Poor sleep is proven to be associated with shortening of our telomeres and life expectancy, worsening diabetes, ischemic heart disease, strokes, anxiety, accidents, depression, and many more things. The obese do not sleep well. More on this in the wellness chapter

- Snoring: causes relationship problems, as well as dry and sore throats, recurrent infections and poor sleep quality

- Sleep Apnea: an extreme form of "internal throat collapse" with dangerous changes in blood oxygen. Afternoon tiredness and drowsiness associated with industrial and road traffic accidents. It often requires sufferers to sleep with a mask on puffing high pressure oxygen into their airways

- Fungal infections: Athletes foot, genital candida, body crease infections.

- Increased absenteeism from work, 72% higher; and school 54% higher [7,8]

- Psychological disorders

- Urinary stress incontinence

- Gall bladder disease

- Osteoarthritis

- Pregnancy problems

- Polycystic Ovarian Syndrome

- Stiffness: reduced flexibility leads to difficulty with toenail care and mobility

- Regurgitation and reflux: abdominal pressure causes gastric reflux with water brash, a nasty taste in the mouth. reflux causes changes to the lower esophagus, with increased cancer risk. Also, reflux and water brash may occur whilst bending to attend to shoes or feet

- Exercise: reduced exercise tolerance, leading to a reduction in cardiovascular fitness and subsequent risks of cardiovascular disease

- High Blood Pressure: hypertension is associated with obesity

- Weight reduction and low-grade walking exercise can substitute pills to control it. Hypertension in turn leads to cardiovascular disease and an increase in heart attacks, strokes, kidney failure and much more

- Type 2 diabetes: leads to lethargy, cardiovascular disease, amputations of toes, feet and limbs, heart attacks, strokes, bacterial infections, fungal infections, reduced immunity, kidney failure, eye diseases, irreversible blindness, neurological problems, paresthesia (numbness), peripheral neuropathy and vasculopathy leading to infections and gangrene, nausea, constipation and diarrhea. In men, it leads to erectile dysfunction at a much earlier age. Type 2 diabetes is occurring at younger ages and is now seen in teenagers

- Obese babies; born to mothers with visceral fat

This list is far from exhaustive. We have a terrible crisis personally, pandemically and worryingly for our babies, children and adolescents.

But anyone who tells you that calorie-counting and exercise will cure personal or societal obesity, is bang out of order. The WHO and just about every major medical website get this all wrong; stating that exercise and calorie-counting help us lose weight, both of which are patently untrue. I do not blame them for getting this wrong, they just have the wrong advisers. Later you will learn why they're so very wrong. Exercise helps you to stay fit and healthy which is great but should never be held up as a beacon of hope for obesity. In fact, quite the opposite; it is cruel, dangerous and humiliating for the victims of these lies. All of this will be debunked later in Diet Mythology.

Our advice is simple; firstly, lose the weight, then steadily exercise your way back to health and fitness. Slowly, gently and when you're ready. And we know that calorie restriction works initially and then fails spectacularly. The whole world has been conned into believing this bilge, in spite of the science.[4] Restricting your calories always fails. The reason; our modern lifestyle has conned our metabolic hormones to guard our fat stores, better than Fort Knox guards its gold. Much better!

WHAT CHANGED TO MAKE THE WORLD OBESE?

The obesity problem is over 50 years old and is getting worse and worse, year-on-year. There is no single cause and no single cure. Monique and I wanted to consider societal changes that influenced the obesity pandemic. We found many environmental changes, but also know that correlation is not causation; nevertheless, this would prove to be a useful exercise. These were some of our thoughts in this process.

Church congregations are now smaller, as are the numbers of smokers, and smoking is a powerful appetite suppressant. As a society, we spend more time in front of the television and value the dining table less. We work longer hours and divorce rates up. The traditional gifting of culinary skills from mother-to-daughter is no more, and as a consequence we cook less than previous generations. Much food is purchased pre-prepared, ready for nuking in the microwave. Small shops struggle as supermarkets flourish. There are new aisles of food wrapped in cardboard and plastic, perfect for dumping in the ocean. Mr. Kellogg and others bring us a plethora of boxed breakfasts, which have long since replaced the "Full English"; a home cooked breakfast of sausages, bacon, eggs, tomatoes, mushrooms and black pudding, usually fried in butter or lard. Butter and lard have been replaced by hideous cooking oils and margarine. And, as you will learn, in my top ten corporate hustles, the advent of hideous foods like low-fat yogurts.

We have cola and other similar drinks, now home delivered, in ever larger bottles, for ever larger kids. At home these were known as "fizzy drinks" and in the US "soda drinks, pops or cokes" depending on where you live. The correct term is Carbonated Soft Drinks or CSDs, but this is rather clumsy, so I shall use the term soda drinks. The sugar in fruit juices is just as lethal as you'll discover.

Over the last 50 years cars are used more and bicycles less; but have our levels of exercise really changed that much? And, how much influence does exercise have on our weight anyway? Our societies have embraced multiculturalism, and the richness of foods available have changed for the better. Forget the spice routes, East and South Asian food is now available on every high street. Seasonal vegetables are a thing of the past. Capitalism has made us materially richer, but has also befuddled our minds with too many pairs of shoes.[9] Modern life has made us travel more, sleep less. Morning larks are in the majority, and bully the night owls into awakening, rising and working at a time that is neither natural nor healthy for them. Our lark politicians from a time of gas lamps, introduced a nonsense called daylight saving time. The poorest countries have both the thinnest and the fattest people, and for the first time globally over-feeding is commoner than under-nourishment, as a cause of death. Fast food outlets have sprung up in every city in the world, creating some sort of brand homogeneity that is not restricted to fast foods. Fast food stores are commoner in poorer areas, where supermarkets are fewer.

Since 1961, we have seen the industrialization of bread production, with additional preservatives, modern wheats and changed gluten composition. The French baguette is a notable exception, that not only tastes good, but is reassuringly stale by lunchtime. We have seen a coincident increase in the invention and usage of antibiotics, both in meat production and personal use; terrifying as we will explain. In our house we have a mantra; antibiotics are only for critical situations. In the UK, antibiotics are prescription only. In countries that sell them over the counter, this is not an act of libertarianism, but an act of serious harm.

We have seen individual behavior change too. For example, the Victorian manner of my English upbringing meant punctuality, respecting one's elders and never talking about money. In the UK, to ask someone how much they earned, was a capital punishment at the time. At school our headmaster was proficient with the cane. Looking back, I can see that discipline was both taught and respected. No snacks between meals or soda drinks were ever allowed. We ate wholesome home cooked food, usually meat and two vegetables. Good fare, cooked by Mum, for which I am eternally grateful. And a healthy appetite, caused by ghrelin, our hunger hormone. Our evening meal was taken as early as possible and formed one of three daily meals. We were taught to eat slowly and chew our food well. It contained all the macronutrients, without ever any fear of fat. The national norm was a Sunday roast, with roast potatoes and Yorkshire puddings cooked in lard or beef fat; and people were thin. Later we would eat toast with cold beef fat spread on it for supper.

On the discipline front, we understood rules, and these were applied across the spectrum of family life. Peterson's idea that we should tidy our room up before we conquer the world is well-made.[10] Since we met, Monique and I tidy up our hotel room. It shows self-respect and respect to the chambermaids, to whom I always leave a generous tip, genuinely appreciative of their help. We make the bed and fold the towels before leaving for breakfast, where we sit and observe the most bizarre eating habits on God's earth. Included in this list of madness is orange juice; the mandatory breakfast poison proffered by every hotel in the world. The thin guests with wisdom are eating the cooked breakfast with fat and protein. The obese and unwise eat the bread, toast, croissant, pastries and of course drink the orange juice. Knowledge is power!

All the changes individually may not make much difference but lumped together they are a powerful force in the march to individual and societal obesity.

POLITICAL CORRECTNESS

It's hard to believe that political correctness has weaseled its way into obesity, but it has. Obesity has fallen off the list of subjects acceptable for discussion at dinner parties, along with so many subjects that were fascinating to debate. I no longer go to dinner parties. I am not a PC person; I'm a defender of the freedom of speech. There are people who want to stifle the obesity debate, utilizing the tactics of identity politics, to push their radical ideology. They have no mandate to speak on behalf of anyone but themselves, yet continue unabated about "fat rights". Their mantra is that people should be able to choose to be fat and happy. Well firstly, sure; happy for a while, until the illnesses start, then in my clinical experience I usually see tears, and lots of them. That's the cold hard reality I deal with.

And secondly, these days there is very little choice in obesity. Babies and toddlers don't choose obesity and a short life of ill health.

I'm libertarian enough to accept anyone's right to be fat or thin, as long as it doesn't impact on me or society in general. But to close down this debate is unacceptable and dangerous; it ignores obesity as an existential threat, not only to individuals, but to our healthcare systems, and our national solvency. And, it assumes that in modern society obesity is a choice. If obesity was simply a lifestyle choice, why have the vast majority tried to lose their excess weight? And if it were really down to personal choice why do we have so many fad diet companies?

The vast numbers of people with obesity and metabolic syndrome, will impact on everyone else. Burn out amongst doctors, fewer doctors, lower healthcare standards, higher healthcare charges, higher taxes and worse still, reduced access to healthcare for all. Hospitals are in a constant state of being over-run by pandemics. This year it's the coronavirus pandemic. And when that's over, we'll be back to treating the medical consequences of the obesity pandemic. Getting thinner and healthier, not only helps the individual, but society too.

CORPORATE FOOD SCIENCE

We are all being poisoned to death by corporate food scientists, working for multinationals in their quest for profit. They work in their laboratories finding the "bliss point" for our taste buds; the perfect mix of salt, sugar and fat. For the record I'm pro-business, pro-profit and for people's freedom to choose. But when any business supplies a product that is a known poison, is addictive and is killing millions of people, we have a serious problem. When we had a similar problem with cigarettes, we did something about it. The corporate scientists know exactly what it takes to make junk food tasty, transiently satisfying and addictive. Our hormones have been secretly vanquished into a confused soup by the rubbish that passes our lips. We can no longer taste sweet, because we have 50 times as much sugar in our diet than is safe, and our hormones don't tell us when we are full.[11,12]

GENETIC FACTORS

The human condition is a complex one. There are essentially two things that influence who we are and how we look; our genes and our environment. In obesity, people will tell you that 70% is genetic and 30% is environment. And they'd be about right. You would also be right if you thought, wow that's a lot of genetic influence. But also, we have 30% to play with.

In obesity, the influence of your genes increases as you get older. At 4 years old your genes have a smaller genetic influence on your actual size (20%) than they will at 35 years old (40%) and 80% by the age of 80.[13] You see, genetic influences change with time, and the environment influences, in both time and space. So being born in Biafra in 1967 during the Nigerian civil war would be very different from being born in the same place now. And, in turn, is very different from being born now in a small village in leafy Warwickshire.

So, my warning is to beware of anyone claiming that eating or avoiding one type of food, or taking the right tea or tablet, will be a cure-all. If anyone tells you this, I can guarantee 100% they are wrong. We only have around 30% of environmental factors to play with. So, we need to make sure we do this well. But it's complicated and it will take time. That's what the whisperer is all about. Getting you in control and making sure you get the knowledge to influence that 30%. And to make you healthy.

OBESITY IS CONTAGIOUS

We know this in our house and see it everywhere we travel. On asking an Irish friend how he was doing, he replied that he and his wife were happily getting fatter together. People in offices tend to get fat together. Is this because they share the same coffee breaks and muffins, or do they read the same glossy magazines, full of hapless lies about celebrity diets? We know that couples share common good gut bugs. Good gut bugs are associated with leaner bodies. We know that we share our skin microbiota with our pets, but they also lower our stress hormones, reducing our obesity factors; so, don't shoot the cat. We know that people who are obese have a lower diversity of gut bugs.

For a plethora of reasons, it is a helpful idea to whisper to your hormones in a group, or as a couple, because you can learn and build together. There are many lessons from this book that will make your whole family much, much healthier, mentally as well as physically. That's why we recommend setting up diet-whisperer groups locally, where you can all help each other.

DIET-WHISPERING

Learning to whisper to your hormones will change your life. We all want to maintain our healthcare systems for those that need it most. And you will feel so much better straight away. You will be back in charge. You will have total control of your weight, as well as seeing instant improvements in your physical and mental wellness.

You will learn which hormones cause obesity, belly fat and why. And that they are canny, and hard to fool. Like me they are truculent and stubborn, and if you push them, they'll resist. If you fight them, they will fight back and win, easily and convincingly. And if you fail to look after them, they will kill you slowly and mercilessly.

No, to beat your hormones, you must whisper to them. In Aesop's fable, The North Wind and the Sun, the sun challenges the wind to a competition to remove a man's coat "It will be quite simple for me to force him to remove his coat," bragged the Wind. The Wind blew so hard, the birds clung to the trees and the world filled with dust. But the harder the wind blew down the road, the tighter the shivering man clung to his coat. Then, the Sun came out from behind a cloud. And the man unbuttoned his coat. The sun grew slowly brighter and brighter. Soon the man took off his coat and sat down in a shady spot. I can remember the very spot I was sat in my primary school assembly when I first heard this. So, just like the fable, we use whispering, nudging and the art of persuasion to beat our hormones. In doing so, we recreate our senses of hunger and satiety, and feel better and better as the pounds fall away.

CHAPTER WHISPERINGS

- Obesity is not over-eating and laziness; believing this, is lazy thinking

- Obesity and long-term medical conditions are a mixture of nature vs nurture

- Nature is our genes; nurture is everything else in our lives

- The obesity pandemic is a truly global phenomenon

- Obesity will cause the West to drown in healthcare costs

- We measure total body fat by BMI

- BMI has limitations in individuals due to racial differences and build types

- BMI is good for comparing the obesity numbers between different countries

- Visceral fat deep in our belly, leads to metabolic syndrome

- Metabolic syndrome leads to long-term diseases and premature death

- Obesity affects 40 million preschool children globally

- Calorie restriction and exercise do not cause a sustained reduction in obesity

- Many organizations still pump out nonsense about calories in and calories out

- The causes of obesity are multifactorial

- Political correctness is attempting to stop the obesity debate

- Corporate food scientists, know how to create the "bliss point" for taste

- Genetic factors play a bigger part than we thought, and one that increases throughout life

- Obesity is contagious and people do better when they form diet-whisperer groups

- Fat whispering involves identifying our fat controlling hormones and nudging them into shape

- Most diets cause a clash between the dieter and their hormones; and the hormones always win. Every single time. Always. The diet-whisperer plan does not

CHAPTER 4

WHAT IS FOOD?

"Der Meunsch ist was er isst". "A Man is what he eats"

1862, Ludwig Feuerbach

INTRODUCTION

This chapter and the next three are the foundations of the whisperer plan. If "man is what he eats" he can only know what he is, if he knows what he eats. And thereby lies one of our fundamentals. When we eat, or even prepare food, we need to know what it is made from. A fundamental part of obesity is not knowing exactly what it is that we're eating. One of the things this book will do, is to make it possible for you to not only know this, but teach these essential skills to your family, children or grandchildren. Or dare I suggest your parents. Science informs us that there is no age in life where exercise and nutrition cannot make a positive difference.

I hope you come to see food in a different way. In the post-war years in the UK, food was scarce for my parents and grandparents. Being born in the 1960s, food was much more plentiful, but we were brought up to respect and share food. For similar reasons many of my South Asian friends are generous food sharers. Sikh temples, known as Gurdwaras, practice Langar; the giving out of some 10,000 free meals per week in the UK and over 5 million worldwide. Across many communities, particularly those that have known times of scarcity, food is respected. I like the Buddhist idea of looking at food, contemplating the work in its production, feeling it, chewing and tasting slowly, with appreciation; the complete opposite of my hospital life, grabbing a sandwich to go! Sometimes a little reflection and contemplation can be a great thing.

Let's dive headfirst into what food is. We know that we have foods that we like and foods we find boring. What we have to do in any food or nutrition plan is to ensure that what we eat is enjoyable. This and myriad other reasons, are why all diets have a quick win and then long-term failure, as the weight comes back. We're humans and humans love the ritual of eating and what is put before them. Three sprigs of cress on a lettuce leaf just won't do it for me. Not now, not ever. So, might I suggest this as a guiding principle. I'm not going to suggest you eat things you don't like. But I am going to suggest that to lose weight, and maintain that loss, we do need to invest a small amount of our time on the food chapters. Unless we know "what it is" that we're cooking and eating, we cannot win this battle, let alone the war. So, stick with me.

WHAT IS FOOD; WHAT IS A MEAL?

For the purposes of this book, and hopefully your future thinking, it is important to know that unsweetened black coffee, black tea and water, still or sparkling, do not constitute food or a meal. For hormonal reasons it will become clear why everything else is food. So, white tea and white coffee, rice cakes, crackers, celery, carrots, low-fat foods, in fact everything else, is food. In this book, when any food, and I do mean any food, passes your lips it constitutes a meal. So, one digestive biscuit with your elevenses, or at bedtime with your cocoa, is a meal. Even on its own, the cocoa is a meal. We do not use the term snack. Snack implies a tiny little something that is not really important in the larger scheme of things. Your hormones don't see it that way. And as you learn to control your hormones, you will come to see it that way too. So, a meal is quite simply any food passing your lips.

MACRONUTRIENTS AND MICRONUTRIENTS

We know that our foods are a mixture of all sorts of things. It is vital to understand the differences. The terms simply mean; macro or big nutrients that we need a lot of, compared to micro, or small nutrients that we need in small amounts. Water is also a vital macronutrient, but accepting we need

4-6 pints (c. 2-3 litres) per day, we'll put water to one side for now.

Macronutrients are the medical names for the 3 groups of food you already know; carbohydrates, fats and proteins.

Carbohydrates are also known as carbs or CHO. You will come cross all terms, and they mean the same thing. When carbohydrates travel around the body in the blood, it is in the form of blood sugar, more formally referred to as blood glucose. For carbohydrates in the blood, I shall use the term blood glucose.

Fats, we all have a feel for if we've seen meat with fat on it. There are also many other sources of fats from vegetables as we'll see below. It is a terrible mistake to think fat = bad. You will soon learn why this is not true. Fats come after carbs and before protein in the alphabet. Why is it that 99% of all articles on, diet, nutrition and health, order the macronutrients, according to the author's bias? Why do they put fats last? Because, they've been subjected to the common nonsense that fats are the baddies. From the mainstream media, to politicians and your own family doctor; they were indoctrinated with the wholesale rubbish that fats are bad.

Proteins are sourced from both animals such as lean meat or fish and dairy products, and vegetables such as chickpeas, lentils, nuts and seeds. I'm going to expand on each of these macronutrients in the next three chapters, as they are key to your success.

Micronutrients are the smaller things necessary in our diet in lesser amounts. Similarly, we split micronutrients into 2 groups.

Minerals; for example, calcium, magnesium, selenium, zinc, iron and iodine that help maintain healthy bones, teeth, immune system, nerves, blood cells and hormones.

Vitamins. The first 4 are stored in fats and the body can go for periods without them. They are known as the fat-soluble vitamins A,D,E and K. The water-soluble vitamins which are easily washed from the body in urine, need frequent top ups as we cannot store them. These are B1, B2, B3, B6, B7, B12 and folate. And last but not least, vitamin C.

NUTRIENT PROFILING: CALORIE DENSITY AND NUTRIENT DENSITY

These are ways of describing the density of calories (energy), or the density of nutrients, in a standard amount of food. In other words, how much energy we get per portion or how many nutrients we get per portion. The macronutrients provide us with our energy measured in calories. If you like we can think of macronutrients having a "calorie density". That is a certain number of calories per gram of food. And this is well-known, the figure being carbohydrate 4 calories per gram, fats 9 calories per gram and protein 4 calories per gram. We mustn't let this put you off dietary fats, as you will see.

The micronutrients provide us with all the things we need to stay alive. The things that allow other foods to be digested, cells walls to remain healthy, vitamins and enzymes to be created or repaired, our bones to grow, or allow us to maintain good eyesight and healthy eyes. Quite simply without them we become ill and die prematurely; so, they are vitally important. They can be measured by comparing the number of nutrients, for the calorific value or the weight of the foodstuff. For example, calories per 100 grams, is a common labeling. There are many scholarly articles on nutrient density. But its importance lies here; we need to eat less food, but make sure we get all the right micronutrients for development, health and life. This comes from nutritionally dense foods.

And if we eat foods that we are intolerant of, along with our good foods, there is every chance that fewer nutrients get absorbed. We also need to consume less food that is packed with calories, but of little of no nutrient benefit; low nutrient dense foods. These are also known as "empty calories", or "calorie dense, nutrient poor" foods, or drinks. A sugar cube is the ultimate empty calorie; it has not one essential nutrient for the body, but lots of calories. And we're all sensible enough not to go munching sugar cubes. Another example even worse than munching on sugar cubes are the carbonated soft drinks (CSDs), "pops" or "sodas". Alas, we have much learning ahead about these economic and health time-bombs. Nutritionally dense food are foods that give you all your good nutrients in fewer calories and examples are;

- Ocean; Salmon, shellfish, sardines, mackerel, tuna and seaweed

- Land; Beef, lamb, venison that are grass fed and grass finished. The "lesser" cuts like brisket and oxtail are even more nutritionally dense that leaner cuts. The most highly regarded being the liver, one of the richest of foods. Eggs are great too

- Plants, fruits and berries; whole fruits and superfoods like kale, cooked spinach and marsh samphire. Potato skins.

- Herbs and spices, including garlic

Calorie dense, nutrient poor foods are for treats when weight is in the stable phase, but ideally avoided altogether for maximum weight reduction in the reducing phase. Examples of these are;

- Refined carbohydrates; pastries, pizza, pasta, rice, potato pulp and breads

- Super-refined carbohydrates; soda drinks, biscuits, cookies, muffins

- Alcohol; especially sweet wines, but also beers, wines and watch those sugary mixers!

Now, I'm the last one to spoil the fun. Socializing is important for health, and I'm not judgmental on such matters. But you need the facts! If you want to cook breads, chapatis or pizza bases, look at ancient flour like emmer or einkorn. This is so important we have dedicated a chapter to wheat and flour. When you are in your stable phase, then make these a treat and when you do, eat them with true joy.

ALCOHOL

Alcohol is not a macronutrient but is gets a special mention here. For many people drinking is a routine part of life, and we all know that it is associated with many health problems. As a drinker myself, I refrain from booze for 2-3 nights per week. And I have a self-imposed rule that I never take an alcoholic drink before 6.30 in the evening. I am constantly promising and failing to cut down.

So, what is alcohol? Essentially it is a toxin, that our liver kindly sorts out for us. The problem is that whilst the liver is sorting out the booze, it can't burn fat; it is preoccupied. It is possible to drink and diet, but the best way is to cut it out until you reach your target weight. If that won't work for you, then look at what you drink. And in particular find out the carb content of your favorite tipple. Mine is zero carbs with a long vodka. I add sparkling water to the vodka with ice and a slice and 5 drops of Angostura bitters. Delicious. Other drinks that you can have are red wine, dry white wine and shorts. Mixers can be "diet" mixers which have zero carbs. The real problem with alcohol and losing weight is that it will turn off your fat burn and the carbs may start to climb. It also turns off the sensible part of your brain and you might find yourself heading for the pizza house! My general advice is to stop until you achieve your target weight, then think low carbs and a few days off, when you get back on the booze. Habits take about 6 weeks to break, so it might be your opportunity to change your lifestyle, whilst shifting the pounds.

CHAPTER WHISPERINGS

- Understanding food is the foundation to building the diet-whisperer house
- A meal is anything that passes our lips, and we now call a snack or sugared drink a meal
- White coffee, rice cakes, crackers, celery, carrots and all low-fat foods are all meals
- Diet-whisperers do not use the word snack; it's a meal
- Water, black coffee and tea are the only non-meals
- Food consists of macronutrients or micronutrients
- Macronutrients are carbohydrates, fats and proteins
- Micronutrients are our minerals and vitamins
- Nutrient profiling gives us the density of food calories or food nutrients
- High nutritional density food is beneficial
- Low nutritional density foods are to be avoided during weight loss

- Low nutritional food can be intermittent treats after weight loss
- Alcohol is best avoided during the loss stage, as it will slow the fat loss

CHAPTER 5

CARBOHYDRATES

"La plus belle des ruses du diable est de vous persuader qu'il n'existe pas." *"The devil's finest trick is to persuade you that he does not exist."*

Charles Baudelaire, Paris Spleen

INTRODUCTION

Many good nutrition books will state that carbohydrates are the only non-essential macronutrient for human nutrition; yet it is the one we eat the most of. And I understand that, because in an old-fashioned sense, our body's macronutrient metabolism can make everything we need to survive from fats and proteins. In my medical school-days, we were taught in biochemistry we can live on meat or fish alone. Both contain fats as well as lean protein. And in fact, the less common cuts are by far the most nutrient dense. Especially the organs, in particular the liver. Again, modernity has turned to lean meats, and not to our benefit. And yes, our bodies can make sugar from fats and protein.

But there is one missing factor. We need our gut bugs to be healthy for us to be healthy. And these healthy gut bugs feed largely on the fiber from undigested carbohydrates. So, we most definitely do need unrefined carbohydrates in our diet as I shall explain below and in the chapter of the microbiome.

I would most definitely agree that refined and super-refined carbohydrates are not required for human health. They are simply harmful. They give our bodies a shapeless form; they round the edges in a way you'll learn to notice if you observe others on refined and super-refined carbohydrate diets. The carbohydrate arms, legs, neck, face, bum. I can recognize refined carbohydrate poisoning at 100 paces. And soon you will be able to as well.

Refined carbohydrates are directly or indirectly, associated with obesity, cancer, metabolic syndrome, central nervous system diseases, heart disease, dementia, chronic inflammatory conditions, dementia, childhood obesity and childhood allergies. In fact, just about every non-communicable disease of our modern era. Refined and super-refined carbohydrates change our gut bugs; the role of disease causation is being evaluated. Some carbohydrates are our most dangerous macronutrient; accordingly, we will spend a few pages covering their most important and deadly aspects. Are they all bad? In medicine there is never a never and never an always. There are some superb carbohydrate rich foods, but you need to know which are the goodies and which are the baddies.

As we shall, see they are extremely easy to understand. Over the years, terminology has muddied the waters. The first concept about carbs is to look around you. Trees, plants, bushes, flowers, all those things in the vegetable patch, and your back lawn are all carbohydrates. Whilst a lawn mower is more efficient than our teeth at trimming the back lawn and a giraffe better at chewing through the thorns, twigs and leaves of the mimosa tree, these are nevertheless carbs. They're all around us; they are ubiquitous.

Our early human ancestors foraged for carbs. Imagine picking your vegetables, fruits, tree nuts and seeds in the wild, to complement the meat or fish that provide you with fats and proteins. Imagine having to crack each nut in turn, to complement your meal, rather than simply opening a packet and devouring the lot. After 190,000 years of doing this very successfully, human eating habits went through two carbohydrate revolutions.

The First Carbohydrate Revolution; 12,000 Years Ago.

The Fertile Crescent of the Levant lies between the Persian Gulf and the Eastern Mediterranean and curling around Northern Syria. Here was the Neolithic or Agricultural revolution, with domestication of animals and planting of large-scale crops and even granary stores and flour. And, as we witness today, eventually turned to loss of topsoil and desertification. The first massive increase in human carbohydrate consumption occurred. This was the first appearance of refined carbohydrates, from flour, in the human diet.

The Second Carbohydrate Revolution 100 Years Ago.

This is the one that we're in the midst of now. In the last 100 years, we have increased one type of carbohydrate in our diet over 50-fold; the quickly digested carbohydrate. Again, this was another first for the human body. The super-refined carbohydrate. We have expected more of our bodies and hormones than genetic adaptation can possibly offer in such a short evolutionary timespan.

Think of it this way; if we plot man's existence of 190,000 years on a scale of 100 years, we would have seen the first carbohydrate revolution just 5 years ago. The current super-refined carb rush would have begun just 18 days ago! Houston, we have a problem; and it doesn't take Cape Canaveral's boffins to spot the problem is our consumption of refined carbs. Carbohydrates are our commonest food type and are also known as our staples; an energy dense, nutrient poor food like pasta, potatoes or rice, designed to replenish the energy lost whilst tilling the fields or manual labor of any kind.

CLASSIFYING CARBOHYDRATES

There are quite simply two types of carbs. Confusion occurs because of different names given to them over the years. Accordingly, we will stick with this classification.

- Quickly digested (refined and super-refined carbohydrates). Bad.

- Slowly digested (unrefined carbohydrates). Good.

Before we look at these types let us consider in general, what makes up a carbohydrate. Think of a string of pearls (figure 5.1). The pearls are units of sugar. In the human body the one sugar we use for almost everything

FRUCTOSE

GLUCOSE

SINGLE SUGARS = MONOSACCHARIDES

TABLE SUGAR; SUCROSE

TWO SUGARS = DISACCHARIDE

GLYCOGEN

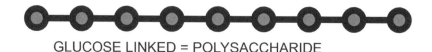

GLUCOSE LINKED = POLYSACCHARIDE

Figure 5.1. Carbohydrates, are made up from chains of sugar molecules. These are broken down during digestion and absorption into the blood and remade for storage in the body.

is glucose. You will note from the diagram that they may be single sugar units like glucose, or two sugar units, like table sugar sucrose. The things that hold these together are known as "bonds". These bonds allow many sugar units to be held together. This is how they grow to make a leaf, like lettuce, grass, or eventually that mimosa tree. The strength of your pearls is dependent on the strength of the string joining them. That is, how resistant they are to the millions of tiny scissors in our gut; our digestive enzymes. It is just the same with carbs; bonds that break easily we call quickly digesting carbs. Any carbohydrate that breaks easily in our guts, can then be absorbed quickly into our blood stream. These are quickly digested carbs. Super-refined carbs are manufactured foods where the carbs have already been broken into single sugar units, saving our gut the need to do any enzyme work at all. And carbs that are strong and don't breakdown into their constituent glucose molecules quickly are the opposite; slowly digested carbs.

Quickly digested; we saw above how these have little to no fiber and are broken down easily by our gut enzymes into sugars and cross into our blood more easily. When we eat these, they raise our blood glucose rapidly and significantly. There are two types and to simplify this further we have divided them by carbohydrate revolution. So, in the first revolution we got refined carbohydrates, flour, rice, pasta, bread and potatoes. In the second carbohydrate revolution we got super-refined carbohydrates like soda drinks, fruit juices, pastries, biscuits, muffins, cookies, breakfast bars and cereals and confectionery. These are generally manufactured from sugar, flour or both and even worse may have added sugars in the form of fructose.

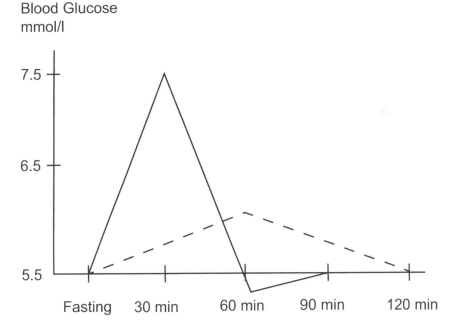

Figure 5.2. Blood glucose after quickly and slowly digested carbohydrates.

Slowly digested; these are high in fiber, less easily broken down by our gut enzymes and cross into our blood with less ease. These are also known as unrefined carbohydrates. When we eat them, they cause a rise in blood glucose that is slower and lower (figure 5.2). Examples of these are whole fruits, beans, lentils, potato skins, cabbage, carrots, cauliflowers, brussels, broccoli, kale and so on. In other words, proper whole vegetables. What mum used to call our "greens". Importantly, these have a different effect on our blood insulin, our fat storage hormone.

CARBOHYDRATE FIBER

Most fiber is found in combination with slowly digested carbohydrates. There is also fiber in a few quickly digested carbohydrates, such as whole grains. Fiber has lots of chains with bonds that our digestive enzymes cannot break down. It is also known as roughage. Fiber has two types.

Solid fiber; which acts like a mini scaffold in the gut. The carbs we have broken down and are waiting to be digested are suddenly surrounded by this scaffold, making its absorption into the blood more difficult. It increases the speed that food travels thought the gut, again reducing its absorption. It is undigested and forms a bulky stool, reducing our risks of colon cancer and diverticulosis. It also surrounds the food with;

Liquid fiber; a sort of gel that also surrounds the food, giving the food an even harder time to get absorbed from the small intestine into our blood. It is digested and fermented by our gut bugs, keeping them healthy and helping with gut bug diversity, which is crucial for mental and physical health, gut health and weight loss.

Dietary fiber draws in water and bulks up our stool, making it move more quickly though the large bowel and produce a stool that is readily passed. It reduces the bad type of blood cholesterol, blood glucose, blood insulin, constipation and transit time as well as many other health benefits, including decreasing the rate of carbohydrate absorption. Fiber increases large gut fermentation, whereby our friendly gut bugs produce good chemicals and gas, which becomes good healthy wind.

A salient point here is that fruit juices have no solid fiber or liquid fiber. They are associated with weight gain and metabolic syndrome. There are no fruit juices in our fridge. Suffice it to say, green vegetable extractions, homemade with our juicer, are healthy, delicious and frequently consumed at whisper HQ. At mealtimes of course.

BIOAVAILABILITY, GLYCEMIC INDEX (GI) AND LOAD (GL)

Bioavailability is a simple concept. Imagine the drug smuggler that has swallowed 50 condoms, each containing class A drugs. If one condom bursts, they die, because the drug becomes "bioavailable", passes from gut, across the gut wall and into the bloodstream resulting in an overdose. So, the drug smuggler is hoping, and possibly praying, for zero bioavailability. That is, it passes out with the stool, completely unchanged.

The glycemic index (GI) of a food is how quickly it raises the blood glucose. In other words, how quickly it is digested and absorbed into the blood. Unsurprisingly, eating raw sugar has the reference value of 100.

LOW GI < 55		MEDIUM 56-69		HIGH >70	
Steel cut porridge oats 51		Pineapple	66	Glucose	100
Banana (not juiced)	50	Couscous	65	Cornflakes	85
Apple (not juiced)	46	Sweet Potatoes	59	Instant porridge	79
Milk full fat	40	Wild rice	57	White bread	77
Orange(not juiced)	36	Rolled porridge	56	Brown bread	73
Lentils	32			Boiled rice	73
Beans	28			Potato/ Fries	70
Broccholi	15			Orange juice	65
Lettuce	15			Muesli	60
Tomatoes	15				
Full fat yoghurt	14				

Figure 5.3. High, Medium and Low GI carbohydrates

It is scored low below 55, moderate from 56-69 and high above 70 (figure 5.3). The concept is simple; give a subject 100 grams of a particular carbohydrate, then chart how the blood glucose goes over time. When you do that for refined carbohydrates you get a frightening chart like this (figure 5.4). So, it actually tells us what happens in the blood when you eat 100 grams of any particular carbohydrate over a few hours.

The glycemic load (GL) takes into account real food in the real world. It takes a portion of that food and looks at the carbohydrate content. It then combines this with the GL of that carbohydrate and expresses this as a number. Low GL is 10 or less, moderate is 11-19 and high is 20 and above. For example, a watermelon and a donut have similar GI at a very high 76, but when we look at how much of this glucose there is per portion, we see that the donut is still very high at a GL of 17 but the slice of watermelon around

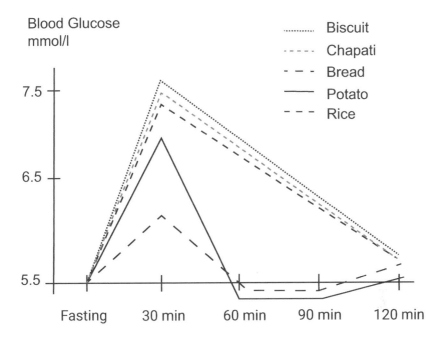

Figure 5.4. Blood glucose afer eating a variety of refined and super-refined carbohydrates. (Graph adapted from reference 210).

3 and is very low. So, you now have an idea of what your blood glucose will be doing per real life portion of each food. In real life, bioavailability and GL change with cooking methods and other foodstuffs taken. Carbohydrate absorption is reduced when combined with fats, proteins or fiber as we saw above.

Spiking your blood glucose is the fastest way to serious, life shortening ill health. The fastest way to recovery and getting your health back on track is to stop this happening. You will learn how to reduce spikes and spike frequency. In that single sentence, you will come to understand how this simple piece of knowledge will give you a healthier and longer life. With even more wisdom we will show you how removing all refined and super-refined carbohydrates from your diet will change your life forever and for the better; on a massive scale. Doing this requires some know how, and we will teach you that.

FODMAPS

FODMAPs stands for fermentable oligosaccharides, disaccharides, monosaccharides and polyols. These are short chain carbohydrates, which are not broken down by digestion in the small bowel. FODMAPs then reach the large bowel unchanged and are used by the gut bugs for fuel. In so doing, gases are produced, and liquid drawn into the bowel, which softens the poop. FODMAPs include fructans, galactans and polyols such as sorbitol or xylitol. In the majority of people, fructose and lactose are digested in the small bowel. Not everyone is able to digest both of these carbs. In these people, fructose and lactose also act as FODMAPs, reaching the large bowel undigested.

FODMAPs are found in many commonly eaten foods: Fruit, dairy products, vegetables, legumes, wheat and other grains and drinks containing HFCS. You can imagine that it is difficult to avoid them.

Some people are sensitive to FODMAPs. This is particularly found in irritable bowel syndrome. The low FODMAP diet has been used to help this group. The results can be dramatic, but this is not always the case. A low FODMAP diet needs to be undertaken under supervision. As it is so restrictive, it is low in essential nutrients and fiber and there may be adverse health effects, particularly on the gut bugs. Once stabilization has been achieved, foods are gradually reintroduced. If a certain type of food causes recurrent digestive problems, then it can be permanently avoided.

CARBS AS A FUEL

Our most common fuel is glucose, and it is the primary fuel for our bodies. Fat can also be used as a fuel and is second in line in terms of its accessibility and its power. Protein can also be used and is third in line. But our brain is very particular about its love of glucose, which is its primary source of thinking fuel. The brain, weighing 2% of our body mass, burns 20% of our calories; some 400 calories per day. About the same as a 45-minute run for a man or 60-minutes for a woman.

When we have not eaten for 4 hours, the blood sugar will begin to fall, and if it were to continue to zero it would result in brain death; so quite serious. To prevent this, our hormones detect this fall and instruct the liver to break down our stored glycogen into glucose. It then releases the glucose into the blood and blood glucose levels are maintained. Our brain remains happy and working properly, thanks to our hormones and liver. Our blood glucose levels run between an upper limit and a lower limit. If the upper limit is breached, we get pre-diabetes. If the lower limit is breached, we fall into a coma and without medical help are dead very quickly. But what if we still don't eat? After 4-10 hours our liver switches to manufacturing glucose from fats and proteins. Once again, this keeps the blood glucose within tight limits. Our brain remains healthy and happy and continues burning glucose as its fuel.

However, if we remain in a fasted state, for example lying in bed with flu, or just a long lie in with no supper the previous night, after 10-16 hours, our hormones cause our bodies to readjust. The vast majority of our body's cells can burn fats for fuel, so OK there. Some 10% of the brain must have glucose, as must our red blood cells and some cells in our kidneys. Our hormones detect we have no new glucose on board from food and kindly ask the brain if it will switch 70% of its metabolism to a new fuel. This new fuel called ketone bodies are made by the liver from stored fats. Our brain is now switched to 70% ketone body utilization. This allows us to go for weeks without food. The liver will make both ketone bodies and more than enough glucose for our brain and red blood cells. We are now comfortably in a state of ketogenesis. This is a remarkably cleansing experience for the brain, washing out all sorts of free radical chemicals and baddies. The only problem here is that we don't cleanse our brain and bodies in this way often enough. We cover this in detail in a later chapter.

BLOOD GLUCOSE LEVELS

We have seen that our blood glucose in health always remains within a critical range. To confuse us all, the units of measurement changed in the last decade, so I'll mention both. The first figure is mmol/L and the second mg/dL.

The normal range for our blood sugar before a meal is 4.00-5.40 mmol/L (72-99). Two hours after a meal it is up to 7.8 mmol/L (140). The importance of having this normal range cannot be overstated. Our hormones maintain this normal range with great alacrity. When we wake in the morning our hormones adjust our blood sugar upwards, so we arise, bright and cheerful. When we miss food, they do the same.

Low Blood Glucose

Hypo is short for hypoglycemia, a term for blood glucose falling below the normal range. Hypos can cause unconsciousness and if severe may result in death. Hypos occur in people with known diabetes on treatment, with both over-treatment and too little food. When people with diabetes on treatments lose weight, they can suffer hypos. So, when weight is lost, there should be physician supervision of medication reduction. In healthy people, hypos are rare. But there are conditions associated with them. Binge drinking, heart, pancreatic, kidney and adrenal conditions can all result in these attacks. The symptoms are hunger, shakes, tingling lips, pallor, dizziness, irritability and mood swings. To a lesser extent it happens in healthy people after eating or drinking super-refined carbs. You can see on the graph that there is a period of lowish blood glucose after an hour or two (figure 5.5).

Next time you're on a ferry or a train for a few hours, do some people watching. When people eat their super-refined lunch with soda drink, soon afterwards they're out like a light. If you want to rob someone, you don't need to drug them, just take them out for a junk food lunch. And when the doctor sees people complaining they're always tired, they go through the standard diagnostic list; tablets, anemia, thyroid, sleep apnea etc. Often omitted from that list, is carbohydrate fatigue.

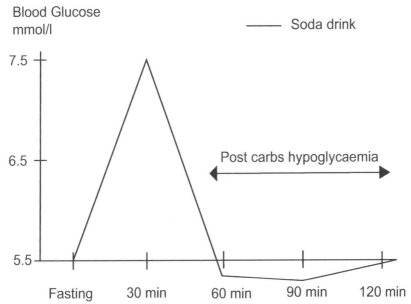

Figure 5.5. High blood glucose falling to suboptimal (hypo) after high GI carbs, refined or super-refined.

High Blood Glucose.

The importance of this cannot be overstated. We have a well-trodden pathway, which goes like this; a diet high in refined and super-refined carbs, then obesity, then insulin resistance, then high blood glucose, then metabolic syndrome and then type 2 diabetes. On your way to the grim reaper, you will have the pleasure of visiting most hospital departments. This will be a part of your life. High blood sugar levels are associated with very nasty inflammatory and atherogenic (furring up) changes in blood vessels all over the body. Not only is this associated with heart attacks and strokes, but kidney failure, blindness, peripheral ulceration, infection and lower limb amputation. The eye diseases lead to visual dysfunction and blindness in many. In the first two decades after diagnosis of diabetes, more than half of all sufferers have eye disease. So, high blood sugar is not to be sniffed at.

The great news is that losing weight can reverse metabolic syndrome. In some people with type 2 diabetes, it can go into full remission. And even if the diabetes persists, it will be much better controlled, and complications deferred and or reduced in severity. As you steadily improve your knowledge you will gain the skills to take back control of your blood glucose, your weight and your health.

Artificial Sweeteners

Note that all zero calorie drinks have the sugar replaced with artificial sweeteners. There is growing evidence that these are just as bad, but for other reasons. They may affect our gut microbiome adversely. They have known to be associated with cardiovascular disease, strokes and obesity. So sorry, they screw you up too.

CHAPTER WHISPERINGS

- Carbohydrates, CHO and carbs are all interchangeable terms

- Blood sugar and blood glucose are interchangeable terms

- Carbohydrates are stored as long chains called glycogen

- Carbohydrates along with fats and proteins are our three macronutrients

- Carbohydrates like all macronutrients' are like a string of pearls. Broken down to the constituent glucose during digestion

- Carbohydrate storage remakes glucose into strings of pearls, called glycogen

- Carbohydrates are ubiquitous in nature

- Slowly digested unrefined carbohydrates, or fiber, are an essential nutrient for our gut bugs and gut health and in turn our heath

- Carbohydrates are two types; quickly digested (high GI; refined and super-refined; bad) and slowly digested (low GI; unrefined; good)

- The first carbohydrate revolution introduced refined carbohydrates, 12,000 years ago

- The second carbohydrate revolution introduced super-refined carbohydrates just 100 years ago

- Refined and super-refined carbohydrates have increased 50-fold in our diets over 100 years

- Carbohydrates have increased in our diets since agriculture began in the Fertile Crescent

- The glycemic index (GI) of carbohydrates

- The body's hormones maintain a base level of glucose in our blood

- We have carbohydrate stores of 500 grams of glycogen in our livers and muscles

- Glycogen runs out after 45-90 minutes of exercise or not eating after 10 hours

- When we have no carbohydrate stores, glucose is manufactured from fats

- Our brain switches to 70% ketones in a fasting state and is cleansed by this process

- We can stay safely in a ketogenic state for days or weeks with 2-3 liters of fluids daily

- High consumption of refined and super-refined high GI carbohydrates, leads to obesity metabolic syndrome, insulin resistance and diabetes

- Insulin resistance leads to diabetes, cardiovascular disease and many other serious problems

- Fiber is essential and increases gut microbiome diversity and improves · gut health and mental and physical health and well-being

- High blood glucose comes with very bad health consequences in the long term

- With knowledge, you will be back in control of your carbohydrates and blood sugar

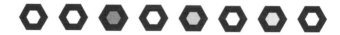

FATS ARE ALSO LINKED IN CHAINS

FATS

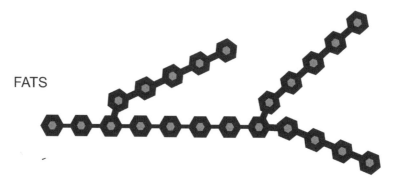

STORED FATS LINKED = TRIGLYCERIDE

Figure 6.1. Fats, are chains, broken down for digestion and absorbed into our lymph and blood. They are stored as new chains, with branches in our fat stores.

CHAPTER 6

FATS

*" A misconception, remains a misconception, even when it is shared by the major-
ity of people."*

Leo Tolstoy

INTRODUCTION

Let's get two facts right out there straight away; facts that are worth repeating
until you are relieved of your own misconceptions about fat. Firstly, fats in
food do not make you fat, nor do they make you ill. And secondly, low-fat
foods do not make you thin. They make you fat because perfectly healthy
and essential fats have been replaced with super-refined carbohydrates. Fats
are nutritious foods and fats do not make you ill; refined carbohydrates
make you ill and super-refined carbohydrates make you *iller*! Feel free
to read this sentence as often as you like. Many years ago, when I first
came across this fact, it made me quite angry. In fact, I'm still quite peeved
writing it. We have been fed this fat is bad drivel for years. The naïve and
the corrupt have been telling us that perfectly natural animal and plant fats
are bad. And it's just plain wrong and in some cases wicked.

Fats are our major energy storage macronutrient, and they are, similarly
to carbohydrates, comprised of long chains of fats, linked together (figure
6.1). Like carbs, they are taken from our blood stream after eating and
stored in fat cells at the behest of the hormone insulin. Fat is our friend
and a healthy macronutrient as you'll see. The exception to the rule is the
man-made trans fats; they are absolute killers and should be avoided at all
costs. Trans fats are banned in most countries in the world. The UK has a
voluntary code, which means for scurrilous owners of takeaways, no code
at all. They continue legally to pedal this poison. In your country, google

it and find out; you may be shocked. We classify our fats into five groups;

1. Saturated

2. Mono-unsaturated

3. Poly-unsaturated

4. Cholesterol

5. Trans fats, otherwise known as partially hydrogenated fats

For the scientifically inquisitive, the saturated chains of saturated fats have no double bonds, whilst the mono-unsaturated have one and the poly-unsaturated more than one.

SATURATED FATS (SF)

These have been vilified for the past 50 years. They were reduced in the Western diet at the behest of the US department of food and nutrition. One thing is for sure, by cutting these out and replacing them with carbohydrates, we have got fatter and more chronically ill. These are the fats found in meat, dairy whole milk and butter, cheese, dark chicken, chicken breast skin, lard and oils such as coconut and palm. The American Heart Association (AMA) currently recommends a maximum of 6% of daily diet comes from saturated fats; about 13 grams, or 120 of your 2000 average calories per day. So, these fats can be enjoyed as part of a healthy balanced diet.

MONOUNSATURATED FATTY ACIDS (MUFAS)

There are 13 of these in the diet with oleic acid comprising about 90%. Most extra virgin olive oils have 85% MUFAs. Extra virgin olive oils are made from the cold pressed juice from olives, without heating. There is a mass of evidence of the health benefits of MUFAs, particularly when replacing carbohydrates and saturated fats in the diet with them. Benefits include reduced blood pressure, lowered bad cholesterol, and increased vitamin E levels. High oleic acid has been linked with good changes in insulin sensitivity in normal subjects and people with diabetes. Observational studies have found reductions in breast cancer risk. People on the Mediterranean diet, which is rich in MUFA's, have shown reduced bad cholesterol. MUFAs are also associated with reduced inflammatory markers, implicated in so many chronic illnesses from cancer and arthritis to cardiovascular disease and aging. They also reduce inflammation within fat cells.[14,15,16,17] MUFAs are founds in olive oil, olives, avocados and nuts such as, macadamias, pecans and almonds. But, be warned. There is a vast difference between the quality of cooking oils and olive oils. Checking your source is worthwhile, as dilutions with cheap oils rich in inflammatory omega-6s is sadly not uncommon.

POLYUNSATURATED FATTY ACIDS (PUFAS)

I won't pretend that this is anything other than my favorite bit about fats in our food. Since I gave my first lecture in Switzerland on this subject in 2010, it has been a source of fascination. Firstly, the terminology; polyunsaturated fatty acids are known as PUFAs. There are three types know as omega-9, omega-6 and omega-3. You will also see them written down by the Greek letter omega, so Ω-9, Ω-6 and Ω-3 and in some literature as n-9, n-6 and n-3. You pays your money, you takes your choice. I will for now ignore Ω-9, mainly oleic acid and discusses above under MUFAs. This section has some real gems about how these fats influence our bodies. Firstly, some facts about PUFAs;

Omega-3 and omega-6 are "essential" dietary fats; our body cannot make them. Both omega-3 and omega-6 are essential for our overall health

- Omega-6s are pro-inflammatory

- Omega-3s are anti-inflammatory

- Omega-6s and omega-3s compete for the same enzyme to be activated

- The importance lies in the ratio, or balance between them in your weekly food; what we call the omega-6 to omega-3 ratio; or 6/3 ratio

- It is possible to measure your ratio by looking at cell membranes and seeing the ratio there

- When you take non-steroidal "anti-inflammatory" drugs they work to block the omega-6 pathways in your body

We know the majority of modern illnesses have an inflammatory component. Common sense points us to the obvious question. What was the ratio 100 years ago, and what is it now? The shocking answer to this question is in our distant ancestors, the ratio was 1/1. In our relatives just 100 years ago it was 2.5/1 and now in the worst Western diets the 6/3 ratio is 50/1. That means for every anti-inflammatory omega-3 in our diet, we have 50 pro-inflammatory omega-6s. That is a staggering figure; the killer super-refined carbs have increased 100-fold, and the omega-6/3 ratio 20-fold in the worst modern foods. With a little understanding, you can alter this ratio in your favor.

This high omega-6 to omega-3 ratio is associated with; [17,18,19,20,21,22]

- Increased asthma; reducing the ratio to 5/1 improves asthma; 10/1 makes it worse

- Increased arthritis inflammation

- Increased mortality in breast cancer

- Increased cardiovascular disease at ratios over 4/1

- Increased platelet aggregation, making blood too sticky and clot prone

- Increased cancer risks

- Increased inflammation in chronic renal disease

- Increased inflammation in sepsis

- Increased inflammation in acute pancreatitis

- Increased inflammation in peripheral vascular disease

- Increased obesity

- Increased inflammatory bowel disease

- Increased autoimmune disease

- Increased insulin resistance

- Increased metabolic syndrome and type II diabetes

- Increased chronic inflammatory diseases

- Increased vaginal inflammatory conditions

- Increased and worsened dry eye disease

I don't imagine blurred vision from dry eyes would have been useful in our distant ancestors. It is a disease of omega-6 overload. It is a disease of super-refined and refined carbohydrate overload. As with most diseases in the list above, a high 6/3 ratio combined with refined and super-refined carbs, proves to be very damaging. This list is far from exhaustive but gets the message over loud and clear. So, the science backs up the logic that we should rebalance our ratios as low as we can, and to aim for an omega-6/3 ratio of 4/1 or below.

Names of PUFAs

Omega-3s are ALA, EPA and DHA. (alpha-linoleic acid; eicosapentaenoic acid and docosahexaenoic acid). In the body ALA can be converted into EPA and then DHA, so is technically the only essential PUFA. However, as less than 20% is converted, consuming EPA and DHA in food is necessary to increase levels. Omega-6s are linoleic acid and arachidonic acid.

Sources of Omega-3s

Oily fish are the best source as well as cod liver oil. Mackerel, salmon, herring, sardines and anchovies are the richest sources. A small caveat for salmon is that their thousand-mile swim back to their spawning ground, is all done without feeding and is the ultimate example of the endurance athlete burning fat. Consequently, they have more muscle and less fat by the time they get home, allowing them to jump upstream. So, the most fats are found in the sea caught salmon, the river salmon being much more muscle-bound and protein rich. Many anglers argue that the darker spawning salmon if caught should be returned to the water. They have sacrificed much of their fat to get back, so they do not eat well and releasing them seems a sporting thing to do.

For vegetarians there are algae sources for omega-3s that are very good and have many other minerals and vitamins to boot, such as chlorella and spirulina. Their mineral and vitamins contents are quite different and so taking both is an option. Research has shown some benefits in reducing triglycerides and LDL (bad) cholesterol and blood pressure. They also contain lutein and zeaxanthin, good for eye health and used to reduce progression of macular degeneration. They have been shown to increase insulin sensitivity and have antioxidant properties. They have been used as foodstuffs around the world for hundreds of years.

Sources of Omega-6s

We need about 17 grams (M) and 12 grams (F) of omega-6s in our daily diet. We just do not need anymore, and we need to increase our omega-3s to improve the ratio for good health. Safflower oil, sunflower oil, corn oil and soybean oil are the major sources in our diet, so we need to really watch our frying habits to limit the omega-6s.

Ratio in foods

When it comes to food, omega-6s and omega-3s are often both present. So, we need to look at the ratios and can be clear in what we want to achieve. Our ratios should be less than 4/1 (omega-6/3). For men, we need to limit our omega-6s to under 17grams. Men also need over 4 grams of omega-3s to hit the ideal ratio. For daily figures for women are under 12 grams of omega-6s and over 3 grams of omega-3s.

Eating good healthy foods is always good advice. When we eat grass fed beef, we get a much healthier ratio of omega-6s to omega-3s. In fact, the difference is due to more omega-3s rather than less omega-6s, which is consistent with the benefits of diets high in omega-3s and consistent with current science. The ratio changes from up to 25/1, to a ratio of 3/1. Fantastic for all the reasons stated above. The same applies to other meat such as lamb

Food (100 mg)	Omega 6 (mg)	Omega 3 (mg)	Ratio
Sea Salmon	170	2000	1:12
Herring	250	2500	1:10
Tinned Tuna (in water)	9	270	1:30
Tinned Tuna (in sunflower oil)	2680	200	13:1
Crab	80	480	1:60
Cod	80	480	1:60

Figure 6.2. Ratio of healthy foods omega-6 to omega-3. Note how the addition of oil to the tuna reverses a very good ratio to very bad.

Oil	Ω-6 %	Ω-3 %
Sunflower or safflower oil	70	0
Corn oil	55	0
Peanut oil	30	0
Soybean oil	51	7
Canola oil	20	9
Walnut oil	52	10

Figure 6.3. Adverse ratio of omega 6 to omega 3 in cooking oils. Soybean oils form up to 10% of the modern US diet.

and venison. But a word of warning; "grass-fed" is not enough to change the ratio to your benefit; it must be both "grass fed" and "grass-finished". The taste and good health benefits are lost if the cattle are grain fed (nuts) at the end to fatten them up; this changes the omega-6/3 ratio from a fantastic 2.5/1 to a frightening 7-25/1. So, be specific when enquiring about your beef; and if your butcher doesn't understand you, find a new source for your meat!

The tables on the previous page give you an idea of the foods that cause our 6/3 ratios to be healthy or unhealthy (figures 6.2 and 6.3). It is worth noting that extra virgin olive oil has mainly MUFAs and the 15% of PUFAs are in a ratio of 10/1. In spite of this olive oil is extremely healthy. Also, note how the ratios change dramatically from extremely good to extremely bad in canned fish depending on whether they are canned in oil or water. And when you look at the figures for commonly used vegetable cooking oils, you realize that foods like fries, chips (crisps), and deep-fried poppadoms are not only delicious, but cooked in vegetable oils rich in omega-6s. They are simply a way of transferring inflammatory omega-6s into your body. A vehicle, like a bus crammed with omega-6s, heading your way. Ugh.

The greatest health benefits come from the magic triad of regular exercise, good diet and not smoking. Get all three right and your risk of heart disease goes down by a staggering 80%. So, like everything, doing one thing will only have a small effect on its own. We know that people who follow this magic triad and supplement with Vitamin D and omega-3s, get marginal benefits. But, in more vulnerable people, or people with little fish in their diet, taking vitamin D and omega-3s can reduce risks of heart disease significantly.[18]

CHOLESTEROL

Firstly, cholesterol. The bad boy, right? Wrong. Cholesterol is transported in our blood by lipoproteins; a combination of fat and protein. Cholesterol is required in the human body by every cell membrane, in cellular functionality and to make hormones like estrogen, testosterone, as well as our fight and flight hormone, cortisol. It plays a major role in the structure of our myelin, which forms the sheath around the nerves that keep us alive, well and moving. The lipoproteins are classified by weight;

- The bad boy. The low-density lipoprotein LDL has had the most-bad press because of its role in atherosclerosis; the furring up of our arteries. Atherosclerosis in turn leads to strokes, heart attacks and early death. However, LDL should be further classified by size, with the particle LDL-Ps being the smallest and most implicated. The atherogenic furring of arteries is highly associated with LDL-P and another lipoprotein called Apolipoprotein B or ApoB. These explain why 30% of heart attacks occur in people with low or normal LDL. The larger LDL particles are thought to be protective, so we must determine which type of LDL we have. When you get your cholesterol tested, you must request your LDL particulate levels (LDL-P) and ApoB, as these are correlated with a tripling of cardiovascular risk.[23] It is worth noting that high triglycerides (TGs) correlate with high LDL-P and low TGs correlated with low LDL-P.

- The good boy. High-density lipoprotein HDL hoovers up cholesterol around the body and returns it to the liver for processing. And HDL is known to be protective for our arteries.

So, now you know which cholesterol tests you need and why.

Dietary cholesterol or saturated fats only increases LDL cholesterol in hyper-responders, and in these it tends to be the larger less dangerous form. In the same people it also increases the protective HDL so the ratio of good to bad remains stable. Egg yolks, particularly rich in cholesterol, are neither associated with increased heart disease nor raised LDL cholesterol. When our bodies digest cholesterol, liver cholesterol production goes down and when we eat less our liver churns out more from the stores. In medicine there is never an always and never a never. There are some people with inherited familial hypercholesterolemia, with high levels in their blood and may be harmed by a high saturated fat, high cholesterol diet. But the message is still loud and clear. Cholesterol rich foods are both delicious and highly nutritious, like avocados, nuts, eggs, liver, shellfish, oily fish (salmon, mackerel, sardines) and grass finished meat like beef, lamb and venison. Bad foods are deep-fried food particularly in high omega-6 vegetable oils, processed meats and sugary puddings, or anything containing trans fats.

And if LDL or more specifically LDL-P is a problem, then it can be successfully lowered by weight loss and exercise. The controversy concerning statins is beyond the scope if this book, but suffice it to say, not in our house! If you are a normal healthy adult and want to reduce your cholesterol, which in old money means lower your bad LDL and increase your good HDL, then there are very easy ways without ruining your life. I hate to see friends ruining their lives with low-fat diets and statins from their doctors. At least ask them to a blood test to find out what your LDL particles are doing. There is a simple way to reduce bad cholesterol and my top ten tips are;

1. Exercise (if you've been sedentary, walking for 30 minutes a day will do)

2. Reduce weight and don't smoke

3. Reduce your vegetable oils that are high in omega-6s

4. Increase your omega-3s

5. Increase dietary fiber

6. Increase your MUFAs, as per the Mediterranean diet

7. Eat plant sterols, but not with spreads that contain trans fats (read the label and see below)

8. Eat a minimum of two portions of oily fish per week

9. If you don't eat fish, take fish oil daily. 1000mg or 1 gram of fish oil contains 300 mg of EPA and DHA combined. And the daily recommended intake for EPA and DHA are 1600mg for men and 1100 for women. So, 4-5 grams of fish oil for men and 3-4 grams for women.

10. If you don't like fish oils take spirulina and or chlorella, but make sure omega-3 content is sufficient

Then enjoy your steak, cooked in butter!

TRANS FATS

Trans fats are also known as partially hydrogenated fats. This is crucial information because these are the very bad boys. They are commonly found in spreads, cookies and margarine. They are irrefutably linked to obesity, cancer, immune diseases, neurodegenerative diseases and cardiovascular disease. They are banned in wise countries like Canada, Denmark, Austria and more latterly the USA, although America had been reducing use of late. It is thought that all the problems apply to man-made trans fats; the very small amounts naturally occurring are not thought to be harmful.

It is the WHO intention that all trans fats be eradicated from the human diet by 2023. One part of the world, India and surrounding south Asian countries, will find this very difficult. Because of the costs of good cooking oils, trans fat substitutes for ghee have been around since the 1930s and were widely used in a country with massive problems from cardiovascular disease. Campaigns from the 1950s recognized the harms of trans fats. As their use falls, just like the West, they will replace them with cheap vegetable oils. A case of out of the frying pan into the frying pan; trans fats out and omega-6s in.

Deri ghee is made by simmering butter to give it its delicious nutty taste. The longer the simmer the nuttier the taste. Ghee originates from Sanskrit and for many Hindus has mythical Godly origins. Some make ghee from boiled milk and yogurt, whilst the Egyptians, Brazilians and even the Swiss have their own versions of ghee. In Switzerland their "bottled-butter" is used for the browning and distinctive taste of rostis. Authentic ghee, made from butter has been around for centuries, and is the proper way this food should be made as a cooking aid. But, the trans fat version is made and used with ubiquity across India and neighboring nations. Tons and tons used for frying food every day.

In the West, trans fats were used in margarine and biscuit manufacture, as well as pastries and pies. Whilst waiting in the car for Monique, a local fish-and-chip takeaway had a delivery of oil. With the stealth of Inspector Clueso, I stumbled out of the car and photographed the labels. On later inspection I discovered they were 5-gallon drums of partially hydrogenated cooking oil. There was nothing I could do, as in England currently, killing your customers with trans fats is still legal! Shameful.

So, for me if I like my fries thin and I'm very fussy about what they're cooked in. And I only eat them infrequently as a treat food. I like them cooked in;

- New, fresh canola oil, my favorite for thin French fries

- For thick chips, Beef dripping, or goose fat; at a favorite restaurant in Bordeaux

- Walnut oil for stir fries

- Corn, sunflower and safflower oils are banned in our house.

- Never trans fats, from any source; run quickly

- Re-used trans fats, almost the scariest of them all. Run, but even more quickly

In China, there is a trade in sewer oil, vegetable oil extracted from the sewers; no comment.

CHAPTER WHISPERINGS

- Fats are a healthy and essential food
- Low-fat foods have the fat replaced with sugar or HFCS and are a terrible choice for weight loss
- Saturated fats are part of a healthy balanced diet
- PUFA omega-6s are pro-inflammatory and are associated with many health problems
- PUFA omega-3s are anti-inflammatory
- Modern diets mean our omega-6/3 ratio has increased to 50/1 and should be under 4/1
- Vegetable cooking oils are crammed with pro-inflammatory omega-6s
- Oily fish are crammed with beneficial omega-3s

- MUFAs are a big part of the Mediterranean diet, olives, avocados, rich in nutritious healthy fats

- HDL cholesterol is good; LDL is bad

- Any cholesterol blood tests should assess your small particle LDL-Ps and ApoBs

- Cholesterol is positively altered by good dietary fats, like omega-3s and the fat-soluble vitamin D

- Check for partially hydrogenated trans fats in your food. Particularly in restaurants and takeaways you frequently use. Pop in when its quiet and ask them. If they won't show you, move on

AMINO ACIDS x 21

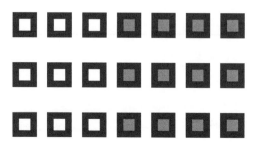

INDIVIDUAL ESSENTIAL(9) AND NON-ESSENTIAL (12)

PROTEIN

AMINO ACIDS LINKED = POLYPEPTIDE

Figure 7.1. Proteins, are made up from a mixture of amino acids, both essential and non-essential. These are broken down during digestion ready for absorption into the blood. From here they are remade into new chains forming new proteins in the body.

CHAPTER 7

PROTEINS

"The doctors of the future will no longer treat the human frame with drugs, but rather will cure and prevent disease with nutrition"

Thomas Edison

INTRODUCTION

Our third macronutrient needs little introduction and is truly ubiquitous. In modern parlance it is "literally" found in every part of the human body. Protos, from the Greek first. In a fashion that is now familiar from our other macronutrients, protein is eaten as along chain of pearls, broken down in digestion so the individual pearls can be absorbed (figure 7.1). This time the pearls are not sugars, nor fats, but amino acids, the building blocks of protein. We can see from the diagram that there are 21 amino acids of which 9 are essential and cannot be "manufactured" by our body. When we string them together, they become polypeptides and when they get even longer, we get proteins. Protein has many vital functions in the body. It is what makes up our bones, muscles, tendons and ligaments. It allows us our movement and gives us our strength. It also gives our bodies the collagen that supports our tissues and skin. Collagen decreases with aging; a process sped up by a refined carbohydrate rich diet and slowed by fasting.

It is required for hormones, skin, nails and hair, and hemoglobin. There is so much more to protein than the muscles we immediately think of. We have carrier proteins that transport lactic acid out of our burning muscles. Ferritin is a protein that stores and releases the body's iron. Protein is used for making antibodies, cell messengers and enzymes. And along with fats,

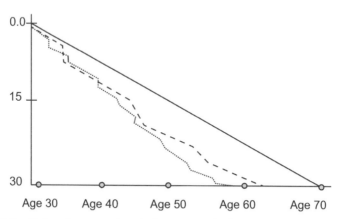

Figure 7.2 . Natural vs accelerated sarcopenia (muscle loss) after age 30 in percentage terms.

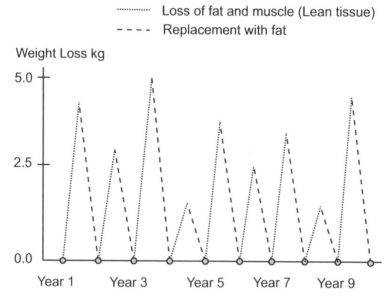

Figure 7.3. Diet failure. The Yo-Yo phenomenon. Repeated cycles of weight loss follwed by weight gain. Muscle and fat lost during the diet, is replaced by new fat as the weight returns.

is of course part of the lipoprotein cell wall. Protein is truly ubiquitous.

When we exercise or do resistance training (weights) our muscles become damaged. Our muscles are subsequently repaired over the next 3-7 days. The muscles must have all 21 amino acids available for those repairs to take place. And remember the "steal effect" that if you exercise your arms and don't have enough dietary protein, your body will steal if from your legs. And vice versa; protein will always be pinched from somewhere else, if your diet is deficient. We all know that muscle is made up of protein, so lean meat is mainly protein. Beef for example is 65% water, 25% protein and 10% fat. No carbs. It also contains many micronutrients such as selenium, iron, zinc, cholesterol and vitamins B3, B6 and B12. There are many vegetable sources of protein too; tofu, lentils, chickpeas, spirulina and chlorella are all rich sources of protein.

SARCOPENIA AND METABOLISM

If sarcopenia is new to you, this can be a life changing paragraph. Our muscles are known as our lean tissue. After the age of 30 we lose muscle every year for the rest of our life. This happens to everyone and is known as sarcopenia. There is little point in talking numbers because our percentage of lean tissue varies from men to women and decreases as we age. The important thing to know is that we lose muscle and gain fat as we age. We lose between 3-8% of our lean tissue weight per decade over 30 (figure 7.2).

As our fatty tissues increase, we get a double whammy. As muscle is highly metabolically active it is a calorie burner. Metabolically fat less active, our metabolism is slowed by losing muscle and gaining fat. This happens naturally with aging but is accelerated by yo-yo dieting; the repeated cycles of diet, lose weight (muscle and protein) and then put it back on again (fat) (figures 7.3 and 7.4). You will see from the chart that accelerated sarcopenia occurs in serious illnesses and shows a similar pattern to repeated dieting. Diets don't work, and worse still they are a cause of accelerated sarcopenia. This matters a lot as a lack of muscle is associated with falls in the elderly.[24]

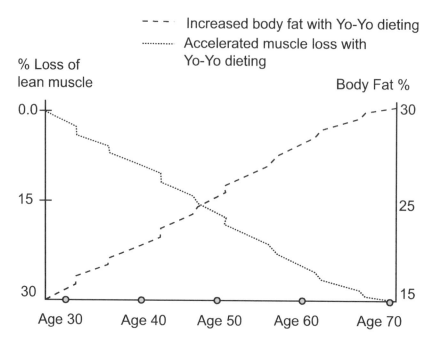

Figure 7.4. Diet failure. The Yo-Yo phenomenon. Weight loss using fad diets is both muscle and fat. When the diet fails, fat replaces to lost muscle.

In the very elderly, falls have the same prognosis as a diagnosis of cancer. So, the message is very simple, build up your strength and muscles throughout your life, and you're never too old to start.

The daily recommended amount of protein is 0.8 grams per kg of body weight. That's 5.3 grams per stone or 0.36 grams per pound. If you want to build muscle, you will need somewhere between 1.2 - 2.0 grams per kg of body weight. That is 7.95 - 13.25 grams per stone and 0.54 - 0.9 grams per pound. One chicken breast is 30 grams of protein. So, for meats you can use this as a size guide. It is possible to supplement your protein, with whey for example, and absorb about 30 grams over an hour. Whey protein supplements come with a scoop that measures out 30 grams for this reason.

This is an important point regarding supplement proteins. There is a complex relationship between insulin and a protein messenger called MTOR (mammalian target of rapamycin). When nutrient proteins and carbohydrates are present in the blood, they both stimulate MTOR to get on with building muscle. When MTOR is higher we build more muscle. MTOR is raised most, when we feed on branched chain amino acids (BCAAs) and of these, the most powerful is leucine. The other two are valine and isoleucine and are also powerful simulators of MTOR and muscle repair and growth. And these supplements are available on their own, usually in the mixture 2:1:1. But as much as these may stimulate MTOR, the real lesson here is that you can only build muscle if all 21 amino acids around.

If you take protein with fats and slowly absorbed (unrefined) vegetables with lots of fiber, it is possible to absorb up to more than twice as much protein. That is over 60 grams from a protein rich meal. Even so, if you want to build muscle then you may supplement your diet with whey protein. This has been shown to have other benefits including reduced blood pressure and reduced insulin resistance in all people studied. It also reduces appetite via a series of hormones (cholecystokinin; GLP-1 and leptin our satiety hormone) and by reducing ghrelin, our hunger hormone. So, if you don't fancy the 5 chicken breasts, there is an alternative.

CHAPTER WHISPERINGS

- There are 21 amino acids of which 9 are essential
- This macronutrient is another string of pearls, this time with amino acids
- Protein is found in meat, fish, dairy, nuts and some vegetables
- Protein and its amino acids are present in so many of the body's tissues apart from muscle
- Our muscles get smaller after the age of 30; a process called sarcopenia
- Sarcopenia is worsened significantly by yo-yo dieting which mimics the affects that severe illnesses have on muscle mass
- We have established our daily requirements for protein and can use an average chicken breast to assess 30 grams
- We can safely supplement with whey protein which also reduces our appetite
- We can and must build muscle as we get older
- BCAAs will stimulate insulin and MTOR to build muscle, but this can only happen when all 21 amino acids are present.

CHAPTER 8

DIGESTION MADE SIMPLE

"Things sweet to taste, prove in digestion sour"
W. Shakespeare. Richard II.

INTRODUCTION

Of course, we all benefit a bit from knowing how our body works, but rather than try to make you the next Christiaan Barnard, I'll stick to the relevant bits, that you need to know; the where and how of food absorption. Cells join together to form tissues and tissues join together to form organs.

THE ALIMENTARY CANAL

That's the medical name for the sewage pipe that goes through you and connects your mouth to your anus. At the bottom end is a ring of muscle that is called the anal sphincter; and a very clever fellow it is too. Thankfully, it retains its muscle tone whilst we sleep, and to my utter bemusement, can differentiate between a fart and solids. With liquids our sphincter is less discriminative; during a bout of Montezuma's revenge, prudence may help avoid that disastrous shart. We can usually, at least in the US and UK, go out for a meal and hold true to the ideology of trusting a fart. Flatulence is a sign of a healthy diet and fermenting microbiome. Enviably and rather efficiently, a dog's anus is self-cleaning. So, there we have it. A ring of muscle is called a sphincter; at the top the lips, and at the bottom the anus, with a sewage pipe in between.

CLEAN AND DIRTY

Eat feces and you get ill. Get feces in your blood stream and your dead. And you don't need a doctor to tell you that. And this is an important concept. Food turns to poop as it travels down our gut. The inside of our gut is classed as outside of the body. Imagine if you hold a hosepipe and water passes through it, your hand stays dry. And that's the same with the bowel, also called the called gut, intestine or alimentary canal. Food goes in at the top, some clever stuff happens, and poop emerges at the bottom. So, what happens in between?

SMALL BOWEL

At the top you have a straight tube that goes to your stomach, the esophagus. Your stomach is a muscular bag, that mixes your chewed food with stomach acid, and then squeezes it out into the next pipe, your small intestine. This is made up of three parts called the duodenum, the jejunum and the ileum. It is here in the small intestine that the food is broken down further by digestive enzymes and absorbed into your blood. The small bowel is 1 inch (2.5 cm) in diameter and is 10 feet (c. 3 meters) long. It ends where it joins the large intestine. Diseases of the small intestine include Crohn's disease, ulcers, celiac disease and small intestine bacterial overgrowth (SIBO). The gut wall has muscle fibers which gently squeeze the food along, a propelling process known as peristalsis. Two organs pump in digestive juices at the top of the small gut, the gall bladder via the bile ducts and the pancreas. As our food passes though it emerges into the next pipe, our large intestine (figure 8.1).

LARGE BOWEL

After our food is digested and absorbed in the small bowel it emerges into the large bowel, just above your right groin. At this junction of small and large gut lies your appendix, or your appendectomy scar! Diseases of the large bowel include constipation, irritable bowel syndrome (IBS), diarrhea and ulcerative colitis. You may also have heard of "leaky gut", whereby poor

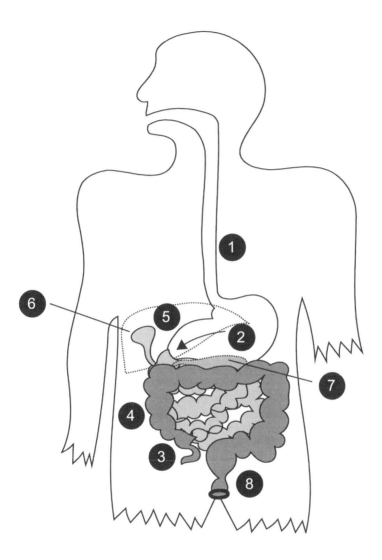

Figure 8.1. 1; Food pipe or esophagus. 2; Stomach emptying into light grey small intestine (arrow). 3; Caecum and appendix where small intestine empites into large bowel. 4; Colon or large gut. 5; Liver. 6; Gall bladder opening into smalll intestine. 7; Pancreas opening into small intestine. 8; Rectum and anus.

bowel health contributes to poor mental and physical well-being as well as autoimmune diseases. The large bowel is 3 inches (c. 8 cm) in diameter and 5 feet (c. 1.50 meters) long. It passes up your right flank, then horizontally over to your left just under your ribs, when it then passes down on the left flank into you rectum, where the poop is in a holding pattern until air traffic control allows it to touch down, traditionally in the pan. In Germany, their bogs have an inspection shelf; disconcerting to us English speakers. In France, just a few years ago it was two footplates with a hole in the middle of the ground; difficult enough when sober. In the Middle East some sort of jet spray is preferred to paper and in Greece, the birthplace of democracy, the outlet pipe capacity allows for liquids and solids but not paper, which must be deposited in a bag. In Japan, they now have computerized versions that play music whilst your undercarriage gets a blow dry. Make up your own mind.

The function of the large bowel is the manufacture of poop from the remnants of digestion. It does so by absorbing much of the water out of it. Again, in the same sterile way that happened to the macronutrient particles. Our bowels contain 39,000,000,000,000 microorganisms, called the microbiome, to which we have dedicated a whole chapter, such is its importance. If you learn one thing from this book is to look after your microbiome. Tender loving care is required.

DIGESTION

Macronutrients as eaten cannot be absorbed. Remember the hose pipe. They would just pass through us like the water through the hose. What we have to do is mash up the food into a pulp, then throw some clever enzymes at it. The enzymes break all those strings of pearls into their constituent parts. So, carbs are broken down into mono and disaccharides; one or two sugar units. Fats and proteins are similarly broken down into their constituent parts; their next obstacle to reaching our bloodstream is the bowel wall. If we simply had holes though our bowel wall into our blood, infection would pass into the blood from the bowel; and that's not great. When Harry Potter was waiting for the Hogwarts Express, he had to get to platform 9

¾, which lay between platform 9 and 10. He did so by walking through the brick wall. And the secret here is that as he passed through, the wall stayed intact. Whilst many thought this incredible, most doctors recognized this as the normal, yet miraculous way macronutrients move from the bowel, through the bowel wall and into the blood. The bowel is our platform 9, the wall of which our macronutrients must cross, to catch the blood express, which will take us not to Hogwarts, but the liver for processing. If you perforate your bowel and the bowel contents enter the surrounding sterile peritoneum, resulting in peritonitis, there is a 30% risk of death. And that's in the very best hospitals in the world.

We chew our food as the first process of breaking it down. It then gets an acid wash in the stomach and gets churned around into a nutrient rich mixture of macronutrients, carbs, proteins and fats. The stomach then churns and mulches it, mixes it will a load of enzyme rich juices from your stomach and pancreas and like a sausage machine squeezes the mush into the small intestine where absorption of nutrients occurs.

ABSORPTION

The rules of absorption are very simple. The longer your small intestine, the more absorption of macronutrient particles take place. The other variables are contact with the gut wall is required, so surface area is a factor. And the speed at which food passes through is also a factor; the slower, the more absorption of food. There are many factors that affect this. Our intestine is not like the smooth hose pipe inside. It has three clever tricks to increase its contact with the nutrients;

- It has undulations, like the ridge and furrows of ancient fields.

- Finger like projections emanating from the gut wall called villi. These are 5/8th inch (1.50 mm) long and number about 10,000 per square inch.

- Microvilli, or mini-fingers emanating from the fingers themselves.

The effect of these anatomical features is to increase the surface area some 600 times compared with a smooth walled pipe.

BIOAVAILABILITY AND FIBER

This is very important. The blood level of our hormone insulin rises in proportion to the amount of sugar, and rate that sugar passes, from our small gut into the blood. If we eat an orange whole, we get a very different rise in insulin, compared with drinking the juice from that orange. Orange juice is effectively 10 sugar cubes dissolved in water. Yes, plus a few micronutrients, I'll give you that. But fruit juice, needing little digestion, rushes across the gut wall into the blood stream and causes a massive spike in blood glucose and blood insulin. It has high bioavailability. When we eat the orange, the bioavailability is lower because the whole orange contains both hard and soft fiber. The two types of fiber surround the sugar making it harder to contact the gut wall, and contact is necessary for it to cross though and into our bloodstream. The fiber also speeds up the transit of the food, further lowering its absorption rate and hence its bioavailability So, this affords us one of the benefits of fiber; less blood glucose, with a gentler rise in insulin and less total insulin required. This is all very good, so eating whole fruit is the way to go. The juiced version is very bad, and not the way to go.

BIOVAILABILITY AND MICRONUTRIENTS

Our ability to absorb micronutrients is dependent on our genes, our environment and the constituents of our microbiome. We are very individual, and so is the bioavailability of micronutrients. If the packet says 100% of our recommended daily intake (RDI) for iron, or selenium, or zinc, it doesn't stop there. The next question is how much will you absorb? If you don't absorb it, your body can't use it. And the answer is complex, because it varies between humans.

SYNERGISTIC FOODS

This is where one or more foods work to aid the absorption or effects of another. These are foods that when combined increase micronutrient absorption or effect. One plus one equals three if you like. Examples are tomato's and broccoli, tomatoes peel-on and olive oil, turmeric and black pepper, apples and their peel, fruits combined like a fruit salad, garlic and fish.

ANTAGONISTIC FOODS

This happens where one or more foods work against the absorption or effects of another, like vitamin A and vitamin D, and Vitamin D and certain anticoagulants.

CHAPTER WHISPERINGS

- Cells join to form tissues, and tissues join to form organs
- From mouth to anus is our alimentary canal or gut
- The gut is both inside us, but outside us
- The body and blood are sterile, but the gut is not
- The gut has friendly bugs called our microbiome
- Digestion breaks down our food into its constituent "pearls"
- Unless a food is absorbed it will never reach its nutrient target
- The tiny macronutrients are absorbed across the gut wall into our blood
- Different macronutrients affect insulin more or less
- Fiber reduces the surge in blood glucose from carbohydrates
- Juicing fruit increases our surge in blood glucose from the carbohydrates
- Whole fruits are a good carbohydrate food, fruit juice is a bad carbohydrate food
- Micronutrients may be synergistic or antagonist to each other

CHAPTER 9

WHEAT AND GLUTEN

"Nobody is qualified to become a statesman who is entirely ignorant of the problem of wheat"

Socrates

INTRODUCTION

Wheat is a worldwide staple food. Domesticated from wild grasses, it has fed us for thousands of years. Our ancestors developed modern civilization, building cities fueled on wheat. It is the world's most ubiquitous crop. Wheat is the foundation of many delicious foods including bread. In-store bakeries have long since directed their ventilation at the customer entrance enticing us in. The supermarket behemoths know that we can't resist the smell of freshly baked bread. Wheat provides 20% of the protein for more than half the world's population. It is a source of valuable micronutrients, such as magnesium, B vitamins and folic acid. But wheat is also one of the most controversial foods. Gluten, the main protein in wheat causes serious disease in susceptible people and the rest of us are worried that we too may be at risk. In highly processed forms of wheat, such as white flour, it is a high GI food and in excess causes serious metabolic problems, as any refined carbohydrate does.

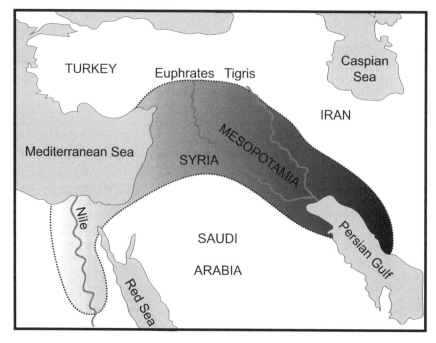

Figure 9.1. The Fertile Crescent in the eastern Mediterranean was the birthplace of agriculture. From there, cultivation techniques spread across the entire world.

THE WAY WE WERE

Homo sapiens traveled out of Africa and soon ruled the world. Fearsome hunter-gatherers dominated the animal kingdom for hundreds of thousands of years. Our ancestors then settled and became farmers; and agriculture was born 12,000 years ago in the Levant. From there, agriculture spread across the entire planet. Animal domestication started with sheep and goats and plant domestication with cereals. Wild grasses were one of the earliest cultivated crops. Wheat grasses were huge towering wild plants: self-pollinating, with small hulled seeds. The grasses were diverse and composed of many closely related strains. Wheat was soon cultivated throughout the world, as we entered the first carbohydrate revolution (figure 9.1).

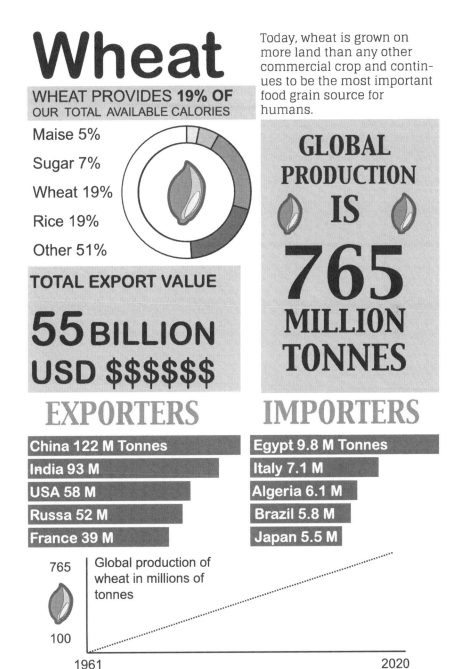

Wheat

Today, wheat is grown on more land than any other commercial crop and continues to be the most important food grain source for humans.

WHEAT PROVIDES 19% OF OUR TOTAL AVAILABLE CALORIES

Maise 5%

Sugar 7%

Wheat 19%

Rice 19%

Other 51%

GLOBAL PRODUCTION IS 765 MILLION TONNES

TOTAL EXPORT VALUE

55 BILLION USD $$$$$$

EXPORTERS

China 122 M Tonnes

India 93 M

USA 58 M

Russa 52 M

France 39 M

IMPORTERS

Egypt 9.8 M Tonnes

Italy 7.1 M

Algeria 6.1 M

Brazil 5.8 M

Japan 5.5 M

765

100

Global production of wheat in millions of tonnes

1961

2020

Figure 9.2. Based on UN data.

Wheat fed and sustained us for thousands of years. Wheat is popular because it is an adaptable crop. It grows everywhere, except in Antarctica. It is easy to convert it into flour, which stores well and makes delicious, varied food. Wheat provides up to 20% of the world's calories (figure 9.2).

THE GREEN REVOLUTION

Wild wheat grasses were adapted over millennia. Natural hybridization techniques developed new strains, slowly over generations. The green revolution in the 1950s was to change all this. Wheat was one of the big targets. New and 'improved' dwarf species of high yielding wheat were developed. Modern wheat was born, a stunted crop, standing a mere 18-24 inches (45-60 cm) tall. The new wheat varieties were genetically far removed from ancient wheat.[25]

Norman Borlaug was the father of the Green Revolution. He was awarded the Nobel Peace Prize for his contribution to feeding the world and the cultivation of new strains of wheat. He is credited with saving over a billion lives from starvation. Wheat, a traded commodity since the 1880s, is of vital importance to the world.

After the Green Revolution, industrialization of agriculture began in earnest. Big pharma and big business swooped on agriculture. The era of chemicals and pesticides began. Roundup is a potent weed killer, which contains glyphosate. It is used before harvest on wheat fields, particularly in areas where conditions are wet. The entire crop is killed. Why kill the crop before harvest? Killing all the plants before harvest results in acceleration of the drying down of the grain. In addition, grain weeds and other materials are controlled. These would otherwise slow down the threshing practice. Experts say that desiccation of wheat with Roundup has been a useful tool for farmers. Good for them; Get the wheat dry! In 2015, glyphosate was labeled by the World Health Organization as a probable human carcinogen.[26,27] Many countries have issued statements of intent to ban or restrict glyphosate-based herbicides.

ANCIENT VERSUS MODERN WHEAT

Modern wheat differs from ancient wheats in terms of genetic make-up, nutritional composition and bioactive compounds.[28,29,30,31] It's not hard to believe this. The plants look entirely dissimilar. Modern wheat fields have little or no resemblance to fields of wild grasses. The history of their development is very different. The grains are different sizes and shapes. The ancient grains were hulled, whilst modern wheat is not hulled. Ancient wheat varieties include emmer, einkorn, spelt and khorasan. Difference between modern and ancient wheat are very obvious to anyone who, like me has cooked with both types of flour. They even feel different to the touch.

The nutritional value of wheat depends on many variables. Location, variety, harvesting, the fermentation technique and processing are all factors that affect the end product. There are many published studies looking at the difference in composition between ancient and modern wheats. Experts don't always agree on the findings, as the studies are not standardized. Nutrients in one growing season may differ from the following season and, if this is not standardized, erroneous results may follow. Therefore, there is some debate about the merits of ancient versus modern wheat. [29,32,33,34,35,36]

There is, however, good research to support significant differences between modern and ancient wheats.[31] The gluten composition between ancient and modern wheat differs. Ancient wheat lacks certain gluten proteins (glutenins) that make bread rise. Due to their differing protein and gluten composition, ancient wheats are less inflammatory than modern wheat.[37,38] Ancient wheats lead the field in the number of bioactive compounds, such as vitamins, lutein and carotenoids.[39] Carotenoids are antioxidants with anti-inflammatory roles, and these may play a role in preventing disease, such as hypertension, type 2 diabetes and other long-term conditions. There is a resurgence of interest in ancient wheat, which is now being grown more widely, and these flours are now readily available.

GLUTEN, WHEAT AND DISEASE

In a small number of people, gluten in wheat causes serious medical problems. These conditions include celiac disease, which occurs in approximately 1 in 100 people. Celiac disease is a genetically linked condition, associated with certain HLA genes.[40] Other types of true wheat allergies occur in 1 in 1,000 people.[41] People with these conditions must avoid wheat and gluten for life. This necessitates a lifelong commitment with severe restrictions on drinks and diet.

There are other conditions, which are less well-defined and are grouped under a term, non-celiac gluten sensitivity. It has been estimated that this occurs in 6 in 100 people. People with non-celiac gluten sensitivity need medical assessment to ensure that they have neither celiac disease nor wheat allergy.[42] Diagnosis of non-celiac gluten sensitivity can be difficult, as there are no recognized biochemical markers. There is much debate amongst doctors as to the nature and the underlying cause of non-celiac gluten sensitivity.

The discussion that follows is not aimed at people with celiac disease, wheat allergies and non-celiac gluten sensitivity. It is critical that people with such conditions follow medical advice and avoid all forms of gluten.

GLUTEN: FRIEND OR FOE?

We live in a world where dietary excesses cause more deaths than hunger. Diet-related illnesses are increasing. Because of this, questions have been raised about wheat. All governments know the importance of wheat, a low-cost palatable food stuff, which keeps the population satiated. People are much less likely and able to riot with a belly full of refined carbs. Governments need to ensure that people are fed and fed cheaply. Rising food prices and social unrest are linked. Removing wheat from the world's table would result in mass hunger.

In high-income countries, the worried-well are fretting about wheat and possible harms from wheat. Celebrity gurus, best-selling books and social media campaigns guide public opinion. The popular press has added to the hype. As many as one third of healthy people avoid wheat containing products. Gluten avoidance is often now seen as part of a healthy lifestyle choice. Paul and I were encouraged to find out more after reading Dr William Davis's book, Wheat Belly.

People are worried for several reasons. We know that celiac disease is becoming more common. People with celiac disease cannot tolerate any form of gluten. We somehow think, if gluten is bad for people with celiac disease, it must be bad for us. We hear stories about people who don't have celiac disease, but whose lives have improved once they give up gluten. The gluten free industry is heavily marketed. Gluten free books and products can be convincing, even if there is little science to support the claims.

Humans have eaten and tolerated wheat for thousands of years. It would be difficult to believe that evolution has changed our digestive systems so quickly and effectively that we are now intolerant of wheat. There is no evolutionary benefit to wheat intolerance. Evolution has not altered the modern gut and not prevented it from digesting, absorbing or processing wheat.

But whilst we may not have changed, wheat has. A shift from ancient to modern varieties of wheat has altered wheat composition. Growing, harvesting and processing methods have all changed and these all affect the composition of wheat.[43] The use of chemicals has increased. It is natural to wonder if all these factors have adversely affected the end product. There is at present insufficient evidence to conclude that all wheat is harmful. However, it may be time to be much more thoughtful about our selection of wheat products.

There are published medical papers showing problems with wheat and gluten.[31] Some papers show the opposite.[33] We know that things are rarely black and white. The medical profession does not believe that gluten is harming us. The general medical consensus is that gluten itself is not a harmful protein, except in people who have conditions such as celiac disease.

WHOLEGRAIN, WHITE FLOUR AND BREADS

Wholegrain flour is milled, as its name suggests, from the entire wheat grain; the germ, bran and endosperm. It is also called wholemeal or whole wheat flour. All three parts of the grain provide minerals and some of the B vitamins. The bran is the outer skin and provides antioxidants and fiber. The germ is the embryo, with the potential to sprout into a new plant. It contains protein and fats. The endosperm provides the food for the plant and contains carbohydrates and proteins (figure 9.3).

Wholegrain ingestion is associated with health and longevity. The Mediterranean diet is regarded as one of the healthiest diets and includes wholegrains. Wholegrains help to prevent metabolic syndrome, hypertension, heart disease, diabetes and cancer and help you to live longer.

Wholegrain flour contains fiber, a critical component of our diets. Processed food lacks fiber and this contributes to many long-term illnesses. Fiber is vital for our digestive health. It also makes us feel fuller for longer. Fiber lowers bad cholesterol and helps to control blood sugar. Wholegrain bread along with other cereals are the main sources of whole grains in our diet.

White flour is made from the endosperm, which comprises about 75% of the whole grain. Stripping the bran from the grain and germ reduces the nutritional value of the grain. 25% of the protein is lost in addition to many nutrients, including vitamins; folate, riboflavin and some of the B vitamin group.

Processing white flour does not stop at separating the endosperm from the rest of the grain. The flour described as white may be chemically bleached to enhance the whiteness. Customers apparently really like white flour! The bleaching agents include azodicarbonamide, chlorine dioxide, nitrogen dioxide and potassium bromate. In the UK and the EU, white flour is not bleached, but this is not the case in USA and other countries. Dough elasticity is a prized property of flour. Bromated flour improves elasticity of the dough, but it is a possible carcinogen. Bromate was added to flour up to the early 1990s but is now banned in the UK and Europe. Bromate is still used in some countries.

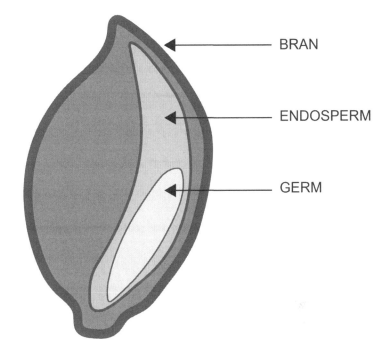

Figure 9.3. Three components of the wheat grain; bran, endosperm and germ.

As the germ contains all the grain fiber, white flour has no fiber. What remains in white flour is protein and carbohydrates. When carbohydrates are unaccompanied by fiber, absorption is accelerated. White flour behaves like sugar in your body and your hormones will react in a similar way to it. Carbohydrates, or sugars contained in the flour, are rapidly absorbed, causing a spike in insulin. You will soon feel sleepy, and you will be hungry in less than two hours after eating white bread. This is a very good reason to avoid white flour. It is a high GI processed food. If you eat a lot of it, you are on the way to obesity, metabolic syndrome and diabetes.

Sourdough is an age-old method of bread leavening developed first in Egypt around 1,500 BC. Sourdough bread is a bread made from naturally occurring yeast and lactobacilli. A starter culture of flour which contains naturally occurring wild yeasts and lactic acid bacteria ferments the sugars in the dough. It takes longer to ferment and rise than other types of bread.

This helps to create its unique texture and flavor. Real sourdough bread is chemical free. Use organic flour from wholemeal ancient wheat, bake your bread and you can be assured of the purest bread available.

The fermentation process improves the nutritional profile of sourdough bread. Flour contains valuable minerals, but absorption can be limited by phytates in the flour. The lactic acid bacteria help to degrade the phytates, thus increasing mineral absorption, or bioavailability. It also has prebiotic properties, in other words helping the diversity of our gut bugs. The prebiotic qualities are dependent on which flour used to make the sourdough bread. Unfortunately, the probiotic organisms do not survive the cooking process. The prolonged fermentation process predigests the flour and consumes some of the sugars. This lowers the glycemic index of the bread, from 73 in white bread to 48 in whole grain sourdough bread. A win-win situation for us and our hormones; always trying to keep insulin, the fat controller at bay.

Fermentation produces lactic acid, which gives the bread its name and flavor. Lactic acid has the benefit of naturally protecting the bread from molds and other bacteria, thus prolonging the shelf life naturally. Sourdough bread can be made from any modern or ancient wholemeal flour.

Fructans in wheat may cause sensitivity in some people. The sourdough process reduces the fructans content and people may find that sourdough bread is better tolerated than other breads. Sourdough bacteria also digest proteins including gluten. Not all the gluten is digested and people with celiac disease need to use gluten free flour in the process. Gluten free sourdough can be made from chickpea, teff flour and quinoa flour.

Humans know no bounds to their inventiveness. The Chorleywood bread process shows us our intelligence, drive and determination. But here's the rub. In 1961, scientists developed a baking method that produced softer bread, at a cheaper price. Originating in the British Baking Industries Research Association in Chorleywood, it has gained acceptance worldwide. We are told that soft springy loaves are what people want. It is certainly not what their insulin or metabolism want.

The Chorleywood Bread Process involves vigorous dough mixing with shortened fermenting time. The dough is combined with fats and emulsifiers, oxidizing agents, enzymes, extra yeast and water. Vacuum is used during mixing to control gas bubble and size. The dough does not need to rest after mixing. Enzymes do not have to be on the list of ingredients as they are degraded by the baking process. Aaagh...

What benefits were there? The process was much, much quicker and less equipment was needed. The process was highly efficient, and the product consistent. There was less wastage, it was cheap to produce, and the shelf life was prolonged. Large scale production of bread was born. People had their cheap soft springy loaves, that lasted for a week. The Chorleywood bread process is responsible for up to 80% of all loaves eaten in Britain.

Bread aficionados don't like this system of bread making as the taste is considered to be poor. When Paul and I visit France, our first treat is a French baguette, spread thickly with butter and enjoyed outside in the French countryside. And I stress, a very intermittent treat food for us! You've guessed it-no Chorleywood Bread Process for the French baguette. C'est interdit.

Comparison of the overall nutrient content has revealed little difference between conventionally baked white bread and bread baked with the Chorleywood Bread Process. There are some concerns about the effect of the shortened fermentation process in adverse effects on the colonic fermentation and gut microbiota.[44]

Ancient grains make delicious bread. They are ideal for flat breads and sourdough bread. This coupled with their nutrient properties, lower inflammatory profile and individual taste make these breads top of the pile. The bread made from ancient grains differs from that made from modern wheat. The higher proportions of glutenins in modern flour give high baking volume. This creates a lighter loaf, something that we have become accustomed to. Ancient grains have a softer dough with poor elasticity and hence make a denser type of bread.

FREQUENTLY ASKED QUESTIONS

Does Gluten Cause Inflammation?

Yes. But most of us are tolerant of gluten. Proteins are inflammatory and this includes proteins in wheat. Wheat protein is composed of three different proteins and subgroups-gluten, globulins and albumin. Each of the proteins has differing inflammatory properties. One of the most inflammatory proteins is alpha 2-gliadin protein, a gluten protein called 33-mer. This protein is implicated in the development of celiac disease. 33-mer is absent in emmer and einkorn but present in modern wheat varieties and spelt.

Can I avoid all inflammatory foods?

No. Many foods are inflammatory. The goal is not necessarily to avoid all inflammatory foods. It is a good aim to reduce the inflammatory load in your diet. A meal may have a combination of pro-inflammatory (e.g. meat) and anti-inflammatory foods (e.g. leafy greens, tomatoes), bringing the entire meal into balance.

Is there a downside to avoiding gluten?

Yes. Consumption of wholegrains is part of a healthy diet. Wholegrains reduce the risk of heart disease, strokes, cancer and premature death. For most of us, wholegrains are provided by wholegrain breads and cereals. Research has shown that people eating gluten free diets tend to have a much lower proportion of wholegrains compared to other diets. If you know what to do, you can avoid gluten and still eat wholegrains. In practice, this tends not to be very well done.[45]

Which wholegrains contain gluten?

Wheat, rye and barley

Are there gluten free wholegrains?

Yes. These include oats, quinoa, brown or wild rice, buckwheat, sorghum, tapioca, millet and amaranth. But be very careful if you have celiac disease - these wholegrains may be grown, stored or processed with grains containing gluten, particularly oats.

Does avoiding gluten prevent celiac disease?

Yes and no. There is no evidence that avoiding gluten in adulthood prevents the onset of celiac disease. Children with a genetic susceptibility to celiac disease have been shown to benefit from restriction of gluten.

Who should avoid all types of gluten?

People with celiac disease, wheat allergies and non-celiac gluten sensitivity

I have celiac disease, are there any new developments?

Yes, but in the future. Providing the population with gluten free products has spawned a billion-dollar industry. There is continuous research into developing a wheat which does not have the inflammatory gliadin proteins, which are part of the gluten protein.[46] Food processing strategies are also being developed to remove gluten from food. In the future, this research may provide people with celiac disease additional food options.

I'm still worried about eating gluten and bread: is there a halfway house?

Humans love eating bread, and it is a pleasure that you can continue in moderation. There are ways to minimize your exposure and possible harms. As the potential problems include the variety of wheat, growing methods, harvesting and processing methods, we need to consider all the aspects of flour that we eat. Consider using organic flour - you will at least avoid Roundup used on the crops. Eat only wholegrain flour; we all need extra fiber in our diets. Eat ancient grains, particularly einkorn, followed by emmer and khorasan. Don't eat white bread as there is no fiber, it is highly processed and has a high glycemic index. Eat wholemeal sourdough bread; it has the lowest glycemic index and high nutrient value. Bake your own bread, you know exactly what is in it, and source your flour with care!

Can I eat too much bread?

Yes. Bread contains carbohydrate, and a lot of it. You should manage your carbohydrate intake based on your needs. Make sure that when you eat carbohydrate it is accompanied by fiber, such as wholegrain rather than white bread. If you eat too much bread, your hormones and in particular the fat controller and fat storage hormone insulin, will reward you with a wheat belly. Your belly will grow and grow. Instead of a beer belly you will have a bread belly.

CHAPTER WHISPERINGS

- Wheat was one of the first domesticated crops and has sustained us for millennia

- The so-called "Green Revolution" in the 1950s delivered industrialization of agriculture with big business, pesticides and fertilizers

- The green revolution delivered new wheat strains with alteration of the plant characteristics, the flour derived from it and the gluten composition

- Ancient wheat varieties have a higher nutrient value and are less inflammatory than modern wheat.

- Gluten causes serious diseases in susceptible people, and they must avoid all forms of gluten

- A gluten free diet, in those who are well, is not always a healthy option. It is extremely restrictive and has been shown to be associated with a low fiber intake in those who follow it

- The type of flour and the bread making process affects the glycemic index and the healthiness of bread

- White flour is the equivalent of pure sugar and should be avoided at all costs. Don't wake up the insulin fat controller

- The healthiest bread option is homemade, from wholemeal ancient flour wheat, made using the sourdough technique

CHAPTER 10

GUT MICROBIOME

"Let food be thy medicine and medicine be thy food"

Hippocrates

INTRODUCTION

You feel human. You think you are human. But your body is outnumbered by bugs. You are carrying more than 39 trillion bugs.[47] They surround you; they live on your skin and in your gut. The collection of bugs in your gut is called the gut microbiota. Your gut bugs weigh in at 5 pounds (c. 2kg) and are heavier than your brain. We have evolved with gut bugs for millions of years. They come in all shapes and sizes and there are over a thousand different species in your gut. We live cheek by jowl in a close, mutually beneficial relationship.[48] If you get this right, you can be the picture of health. Get it wrong and you may find yourself in a perilous state. Like it or not, your health and well-being is dependent on your gut bugs.

WHAT ARE YOUR GUT BUGS?

We carry 1,500 different species of organisms in our gut (figure 10.1). Humans evolved with bugs and most of them are friendly. There are tiny numbers of dangerous ones, but these are held in check by the rest of the pack. A sort of safety in numbers. There are some terms that you will come across in relation to the bugs within your gut. In this chapter, I will usually refer to them as gut bugs, but the accepted medical terms are as follows:

Microbiome is a collective term used for the colonies of bugs coexisting with you. Gut microbiome refers to the colonies in your gut. It refers to the

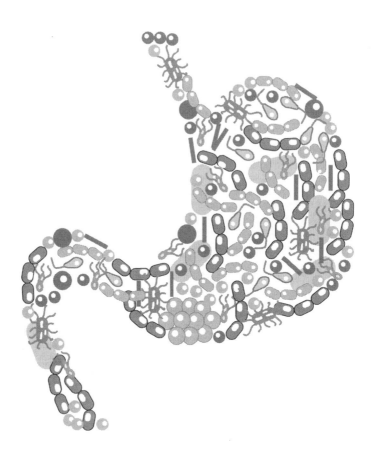

Figure 10.1. The microorganisms in your gut are composed of bacteria, archaea, eukaryotes and viruses.

genetic makeup of the bugs.

Microbiota is also the term used for the bugs, which coexist with you. Gut microbiota refers to the bugs themselves.

Although the words microbiome and microbiota have slightly different meanings, these terms are often used interchangeably.

There are bugs along the entire length of the gut.[49] The largest numbers are in the colon. Throughout its entire length, the gut milieu changes and provides many growing conditions.[50] Oxygen and acidity are two important requirements for their growth. Bugs are very specific in their needs, some tolerating high acidity with low oxygen levels, others needing the opposite. The distribution of bugs in the gut is dependent on the particular growing conditions. Different species are found, in varying proportions, throughout the length of the gut.

The growth requirements of bugs are so specific, that different bugs are found in the middle of the gut compared to the gut wall. The gut wall itself is a highly specialized environment, some bugs living on the wall itself and others in close proximity to the wall. Many gut bugs do not exist anywhere else in nature.

The Human Microbiome Project changed our understanding of the gut microbiome or microbiota.[51,52] It unlocked the genetic composition and functions of the gut bugs. Prior to the Human Microbiome Project, the organisms in our gut were identified by culturing the bugs. Only a small fraction of the species could be cultured. With genetic analysis, new species were discovered, metabolic pathways and functions were defined. At least 2,776 different species have been identified.[53,54] Huge diversity of gut bugs was identified in healthy people. The Human Microbiome Project unlocked many of the dark secrets of our bowel and its microbial contents.

HOW DO GUT BUGS DEVELOP?

The gut microbiota starts to develop at birth. The type of delivery influences the composition of the bugs found in newborns. With a vaginal delivery, the newborn's gut bugs reflect their mother's vaginal and or gut bugs. Following cesarean section delivery, the gut bugs reflect the organisms found in the hospital environment; far from the ideal bugs for a baby gut. These changes can have lasting adverse health implications.[55]

Colonization of the gut with bugs proceeds rapidly in babies. The baby gut microbiota is highly unstable initially and reacts to food, environment and toxins, including antibiotics. The type of food and genetic make-up play a big part in establishing the type of bug colonies. Breast milk contains hundreds of bugs. Breast fed babies have different gut bugs compared to formula fed babies. Both the diversity and composition of the gut organisms increase rapidly in the first few years of life. After the age of three, the bug species composition is relatively fixed for life. With increasing age, at the other extreme of life, the bug community shifts again. And sadly, this is not a change for the better. There is species loss, unfavorable alteration in the proportions of the bugs and loss of richness and diversity.[56]

Microbiome refers to the genetic composition of the gut microbiota. You have a unique gut microbiome. No two people have the same gut bugs.[57] Some generalizations can be made regarding the composition of a healthy gut microbiota. The greater the number of different species, the broader and richer the mix, the better. This is known as diversity. High diversity in the gut bugs is an excellent mark of health.[48,58] A core of essential various species has been identified in healthy people, so-called keystone species. The relative proportion between all the individual species is important, with a predominance of good bugs and a low proportion of bad bugs. Dangerous bugs should be absent or present in very small numbers.

Keystone species are everywhere in nature, including the gut microbiota. The bee is a perfect example of a keystone species. Bees spread nectar and pollen amongst plants, fertilizing the plants and allowing them to reproduce. The nectar and pollen provide food for the bees. Loss of bees would spell the end of the plant ecosystem. Keystone species are not necessarily the most abundant species, but the ecosystem cannot survive without them.

Keystone species in the gut microbiota are amongst the most vital parts of the gut ecosystem. These important bugs hold the system together. Keystone species help the gut bugs to adapt. Without the keystone species, an invasive bug could take over. An invasive bug could shift the gut bugs and us in another direction, which could spell disaster.

A healthy gut microbiota is a stable community of microbes. A core of bugs, all working together, rather than as individuals. It shows high resilience but will be influenced by changes in our bodies and external influences. A healthy gut microbiota is never harmful to us. You and your gut bugs can be classed as a superorganism. Don't mess it up; you may not live to regret it.

WHAT DO GUT BUGS DO?

The gut microbiota does things that we humans can't do. The bugs in our gut protect us, produce healthy hormone like chemicals, control our brain health, regulate our immune system, help to digest our food and produce vitamins. The healthy chemicals regulate our energy control, in addition to many other functions all over the body.[58]

Protection

The world is a threatening environment. We have to protect our self from the outside world. There's always someone, something or some bug that wants to overpower us. Our skin is our first line of defense. Most chemicals can't penetrate intact skin, and neither can bugs. The gut lining is our second line of defense. It has to allow healthy nutrients and chemicals in, keep unhealthy chemicals or toxins out and keep bugs out. The gut contents must remain separated from our bodies.

Our gut is lined with a single, specialized layer of cells. Our gut bugs prevent breaches of this barrier and keep the lining intact. The bugs digest and clear up dead cells, remove mucus and debris from the lining. Gut bugs produce protective chemicals which maintain the junctions between the lining cells.

A healthy barrier prevents both your gut bugs and invaders from gaining access to our bloodstream and body. Dangerous invading bugs can suddenly overwhelm the defenses in severe forms of food poisoning and cross the barrier. If your gut lining is perforated (for example a ruptured appendix) and your gut contents spill into your abdomen, untreated, death follows pretty quickly. A healthy gut microbiota is critical to the functioning of your gut barrier. Failure of this barrier can lead to a "leaky gut". This is more a concept than a disease, but you can see that your gut bugs have an integral role to play in preventing a leaky gut.

Hormone Like Chemicals

The gut microbiota outnumbers humans in terms of gene power. We have 23,000 genes, our guts bugs have over 200 million genes.[59] Genes win prizes, because genes make stuff. Gut bugs, controlled by their genes, produce hormone like chemicals. We can't produce these chemicals because we don't have the genes to do so. These hormone-like chemicals have widespread effects in our bodies.

Brewers add another type of bug, yeast to fermented hops to produce beer. We can't produce beer in our gut, but our gut bugs ferment fiber to produce hundreds of different healthy chemicals. Short chain fatty acids are a group of such chemicals. There are several types of them, and they have a huge range of functions throughout the body. Short chain fatty acids cross the gut lining and are absorbed into the blood stream. These hormone-like chemicals affect all our organs, interacting with them and helping to control our metabolism.

Short chain fatty acids help to regulate sugar processing in the liver. A higher concentration of these fatty acids reduces insulin resistance and obesity.[12] Deposition of fat and cholesterol metabolism are controlled by insulin and the liver, with short chain fatty acids being intimately connected with this process. Short chain fatty acids help in the production and influence the release of ghrelin, leptin and other transmitters, which tell us if we are hungry or full. If we're not told that we are full by our hormones, we just keep eating.

Our gut bugs produce a range of other healthy chemicals which help our immune system and the gut lining. Some of these chemicals are antioxidants. Free radicals cause inflammation and are mopped up by the antioxidants, preventing damage to us. No part of our metabolism is unaffected by these chemicals.

Brain Health

Butterflies in your tummy, a pit in your stomach, and trust your gut. These are all part of our common language; a narrative that references the close communication between the gut and the brain. New scientific developments are showing us just how critical the gut microbiota is for brain health.[60,61] Your gut bugs communicate directly with your brain in two main ways; via chemicals and via nerves. The many hormone like chemicals, produced by our gut bugs enter the blood stream to reach the brain. These chemicals affect brain functions such as reward, stress response and thinking.

The gut also communicates directly with the brain through a nerve called the vagus nerve. This traveling nerve meanders through the entire abdomen, reaching all parts of the gut and then travels to the brain. Messages travel along this nerve back and forth, with constant communication between the two ends. This communication system is called the microbiota-gut-brain axis.[62] The gut microbiota controls messages that are sent to the brain. Just think of it, your gut bugs control messages that go directly to your brain. Where's the free will? Where are you in all this? Who is working for whom?

Serotonin is one of the happy hormones. You need serotonin to feel good. It moderates your appetite, mood, sleep, sexual desire and memory. Most serotonin is made in the gut. Your gut bugs are intimately connected with serotonin production, one of the many transmitters made by gut bugs.[63] They are involved not just in production but bear some responsibility for controlling the amount of serotonin made.[64] Happy gut, happy you!

Immune System

The gut microbiota is a critical part of maintaining a healthy immune system. We and our gut microbiota have many challenges to allow our mutualistic relationship to flourish. The gut or lumen is where the microbes live, and this is technically outside of the body. Our immune system is inside our body. Yet the immune system and the gut microbiota interact and interact intimately. It is a complex relationship, and much still remains to be discovered.[65]

Most of our immune system is found in our guts. Our gut bugs and our immune system start to interact at birth. The gut bugs are critical in establishing the immune system in neonates. Our immune system needs be tolerant of our own gut bugs but also to develop defenses against dangerous bugs. The immune system promotes growth of good bacteria. The good bacteria in turn produce chemicals that support the development of healthy immune cells. Healthy immune cells are able to differentiate between self and non self. Thus, our immune system and our gut microbiota work together to keep us healthy.

The Hadza tribe, hunter-gatherers in Tanzania live a nomadic hunter-gatherer lifestyle. They are not exposed to modern medicines or chemicals. Their gut microbiome is unique, with high diversity.[66] They possess many bugs which are unknown to us and not present in Western cultures. A microbe called treponema is amongst their gut bugs. If you or I were to carry this particular bug, we might develop Yaws, an unpleasant chronic skin disease. Our gut and immune system have not developed protection against this bug. The Hadza people do not develop Yaws and co-exist with treponema. Treponema helps them in the digestion of complex starches. Their immune system has evolved with treponema, which then prevents development of Yaws.

Digestion and Vitamins

More people now die of eating too much, than die of hunger. But it was not always so and throughout our evolutionary history, we had to maximize our food stores to survive. Digestion of food stuffs was critical. We humans are able to produce 30 digestive enzymes. One particular gut bug alone produces over 250 digestive enzymes.[67] Our gut bugs help us with efficient digestion of all foodstuffs.[68]

Gut bugs are involved in carbohydrate digestion, particularly residual fiber entering the colon. We can't digest fibrous foods, such as cellulose, xylans, resistant starch and inulin. In the colon, gut bugs ferment these fibrous foods. Some products are absorbed and used for energy for the gut lining and for the bugs themselves. Some products are used to make short chain free fatty acids; healthy chemicals, critical for our health.

Humans can't make vitamins, and we can't make vitamin B12. Here, we are no different to animals, as they can't make vitamin B12 either. Up to 50% of our gut bugs can make Vitamin B12. Many of the other B group of vitamins can be produced by our gut bugs including B1, B2, B5, B6. folate and Vitamin K are also made in the colon. These vitamins may be used locally in the gut, rather than elsewhere in the body and provide help in maintaining protection of the gut and our immune system.[69,70]

HOW DO THE GUT BUGS BEHAVE?

Our gut bugs live in a community, composed of hundreds of different species. The different species are highly dependent on each other. Many of the chemicals produced by one bug are food for another bug, which provides food for another bug and so on. The richness and diversity of the species mix confers resilience.[71] If one species is missing, another can step in and compensate.

Bugs produce gases during the fermentation process. Gases need to be cleared from the gut, otherwise you would explode. A fart contains 5-375ml of gases, and you can produce up to one and a half liters per day; rejoice knowing your gut bugs are working hard for you. Some people produce particular stinkers, smelling of rotten eggs. You can blame this on their particular cocktail of gut bugs, which are producing hydrogen sulfide. Your gut bugs make up about a third of your poop, about 200 billion of them; many of them alive and kicking.

The gut microbiota like to sleep.[72] Yes, that's right, like you and everyone else, they sleep. Bugs don't sleep like humans, as they don't have nervous systems, but they do have circadian rhythms. Their behavior is tuned to the 24-hour day-night cycle. The activity of your gut bugs rises and falls with you. For once in this relationship, we have the upper hand and dictate when to sleep. It's really quite pleasing to think that as you settle into bed for a good night's sleep, your 37 trillion gut bugs settle down for the night with you.[73,74,75]

All is not quiet in the hours of darkness in your gut. I was reminded of this when we visited Singapore. Going out for a run at dawn, hoping to see the sun rise and thinking that I would be alone, I found that I was wrong. The city was being refreshed, machines cleaned the streets, barges cleaned the lagoon and an army of workers cleaned the bridges. And so, it is in your gut. The shift workers emerge. The night-time workers emerge, detoxifying and cleaning your gut. As the day dawns, they disappear, like the Singaporean cleaning army, into the shadows.[75]

THE GUT MICROBIOTA IN ILLNESS: DYSBIOSIS

Dysbiosis means that the gut microbiota is imbalanced.[76] The most consistent finding in dysbiosis is a loss of diversity of the gut bugs. The rich mix of different species is lost. Keystone species are lost. This allows bad organisms to proliferate and dominate. The vital functions of the gut microbiota including protection, digestion, immunity and brain health are adversely affected. Bad organisms damage the gut lining and promote inflammation. This has a range of adverse effects on us. There are recognized changes to the gut microbiota in many long-term conditions. We do not yet fully understand the role of gut bugs in disease; these are known unknowns. We are getting much closer to a better understanding of the role of gut bugs in disease.[77]

Clostridium Difficile Colitis

Clostridium difficile colitis is an example of extreme dysbiosis caused by antibiotics. Following certain antibiotics there is proliferation of Clostridium difficile, which is a dangerous bug. It is a gut bug colonizer, but it is usually held in check by the good bugs. Due to loss of good bugs, usually due to antibiotic usage, clostridium proliferates. It releases toxins which damage the lining of the colon. The condition can be life threatening.

Treatment was often hopeless with many relapses. Newer treatments with fecal transplants, to replace the normal gut bugs that have been lost, have been very effective in managing this serious condition.

Obesity

There is a famous experiment that heralded huge international interest in gut bugs and their role in obesity. Lean mice were given fecal microbiota transplants (i.e. gut bugs) either from fat mice and or lean mice. The mice receiving transplants from fat mice became obese and the mice who received transplants from lean mice stayed lean. Pictures of one fat mouse and one lean mouse went viral. On the internet, fecal transplants were hailed as a potential cure for obesity. As you can imagine, it is not that simple, otherwise the obesity pandemic would be over. Obesity is a complicated problem, with no single cause and at present fecal transplantation is not a cure.

Obese people have a characteristic profile of their gut bugs.[78] You can predict obesity by the composition of gut bugs. In obesity, there is loss of diversity of the gut bugs. Obese people therefore have a smaller number of overall genes in their gut bugs, than do lean people. The lower the number of genes in your gut bugs, the higher the likelihood of becoming more obese over the next ten years.[79]

The composition of your gut bugs affects the results of dieting. We are only too aware that rebound weight gain, after dieting is a universal finding.[80] Weight rebounds are more marked in people with the lowest diversity of their gut bugs. Those obese people with high levels of good bugs such as Akkermansia have more sustainable weight loss after diets.[81]

A shift in the proportions of different species occurs in obesity. Good bugs decrease and bad bugs increase. Species loss and change of bug ratios alters the normal functions of the gut bugs. There are profound effects on the gut lining, the immune system and metabolism. Good chemicals, the short chain free fatty acids decline. The bad bugs, now unchecked produce unhealthy chemicals, which cause widespread inflammation. These chemical changes are in turn associated with many long-term conditions including high cholesterol, hypertension, diabetes and cancer.

Keystone species are absent or grossly reduced in obese people. Not just are keystone species lost, but other good bugs are reduced or lost as well. Christensenella is rarely found in the gut bugs of obese people. It limits fat accumulation and is associated with normal blood fats. It is a useful bug to have.

While a certain percentage of obese people are indeed metabolically normal, the majority sadly will develop so called non-communicable diseases; hypertension, high cholesterol, metabolic syndrome, diabetes, heart disease, cancer, the list goes on. Body positivity is now mainstream. The fat acceptance movement, a social justice movement would have us believe that obesity is something to be celebrated. This is patently a falsehood. A look at their impoverished gut bugs and all the associated problems might just change their minds.

Obesity does not mean that all is lost. Quite the opposite. If you restore metabolic harmony and lose weight, the gut bugs changes are reversible, and you can restore normal gut bugs.[82] Good species reappear, the ratios between good and bad bugs return. Happy days.

Non-communicable Diseases and Mental Health

Dysbiosis with poor bug diversity, has been found in many non-communicable diseases. These diseases include, diabetes, inflammatory bowel disease, cancer, arthritis and cardiovascular diseases such as hypertension.[58]

Dysbiosis drives inflammation in the gut. Inflammation degrades the gut lining and increases gut permeability. Critical metabolic functions are altered, and widespread inflammation follows. There is increasing evidence that dysbiosis is driving non-communicable diseases.[60] Research is focused on this problem with evaluation of altering the composition of the gut microbiota to manage these conditions. What we really need to do is ensure that dysbiosis doesn't happen. Wouldn't it be so much better to prevent dysbiosis rather than to treat it? We need to prevent these problems rather than treat them. Lifestyle and diet are the key to prevention.

Messages between the gut and brain are continually exchanged via nerves and chemicals. Gut dysbiosis is associated with psychiatric disorders. Links have been found between dysbiosis and autism, schizophrenia, anxiety, stress and depression.[61]

Prozac is the most widely used antidepressant drug. One in ten people in America take antidepressants. In the UK, in 2018, 70.9 million prescriptions were given compared with 36 million prescriptions in 2008.[83] Prozac increases the availability of serotonin. Your gut bugs help to make serotonin from tryptophan. Tryptophan cannot be made in the body. You need to eat it. It is found in salmon, eggs, poultry, spinach, seeds, nuts, milk and soy. If you do not have the essential tryptophan, serotonin will not be made. Serotonin production is increased during times of fasting. If you snack frequently and there are no periods of fasting during the day, your serotonin production will be reduced.

A new discipline called psychobiotics describes the use of the gut microbiota to help mental health.[84] There is some evidence that manipulation of gut bugs is of benefit in psychiatric disorders.[85] This is a very new science, and we will know a lot more in the future. Hippocrates is credited with the following "All disease begins in the gut", but how did he know? Hippocrates may have been wiser than we could have ever imagined.

WHAT AFFECTS GUT BUGS?

Diet

Diet has a profound effect on the gut microbiota. Some foods confer significant benefit to your gut bugs. Conversely, other foods have adverse effects on the gut bugs. Changes to the gut bugs can occur within days of changing diet. A study showed remarkable differences, when Americans and rural Africans switched diets.[86] Good bugs increased in the Americans, producing healthy chemicals after only two weeks. If diets subsequently revert, the gut bugs also revert to the original state.

The ratio of good to bad bugs changes depending on the food that we eat.

If the proportions of gut bugs change, the function of the gut microbiota is altered. It is possible to encourage good bugs to proliferate. It is also possible to encourage bad bugs to proliferate.

Remember the film 'Super Size Me'? Morgan Spurlock ate junk food, specifically McDonald's food for 30 days. This was accompanied by weight gain, elevation of his cholesterol and abnormal liver function tests. Professor Tim Spector repeated this experiment with the help of his son, with the aim of evaluating changes in the gut bugs. His son's gut bugs were compared before and after a ten day 'feast' of junk food. The results were impressive. There was loss of richness and diversity with loss of 40% of the previously detected species, a doubling of the bad species, and a 45-50% loss of two friendly species. Overall diversity had disappeared. Returning to his previous healthy diet, his gut bugs slowly normalized.[67]

People who eat a high fiber diet have a different gut microbiota than people who eat a low fiber diet. A high fiber diet is associated with a rich and diverse gut microbiota. The converse applies, with a low fiber diet being associated with low diversity. On average, we don't eat enough fiber, the average fiber consumption per day in high-income countries is less than 20gms per day.[87] The recommended intake is 30gms per day. Traditional rural communities eat as much as 50-100gms per day.

A refined or super-refined carbohydrate diet is associated with a low fiber diet. These diets cause proliferation of bad bugs. The high sugar creates increased acidity, and this coupled with a lack of fiber starves your good bacteria of nutrients.

A good diet for your gut bugs includes a wide range of diverse foods, in particular a wide range of plants. Diversity with high fiber is the key. Eat vegetables, wholegrains, fruit, nuts, seeds, fermented foods, proteins and fats. A Mediterranean type diet is one of the best options. The more vegetables that you consume, the more diverse your gut bugs.

Exercise

We all know that exercise is good for us. We all agree that exercise improves your heart and your muscles and lengthens your lifespan. It is a little easier for everyone now that we are also agreed on how much exercise to do. We need to spend 150 minutes of moderate activity per week. But your gut bugs? Could exercise also be good for your gut bugs? Could they really need to go for a run?

As an amateur triathlete, I was really pleased to discover that my gut bugs need to run. But I was perplexed how exercise and gut bugs were related. It turns out that the chemicals and hormones produced during exercise have a positive effect on our gut bugs.[67] Exercise increases diversity and richness in our gut bugs. The ratio of good to bad bugs is increased.

Akkermansia muciniphila, a cleaner and vital maintainer of our gut lining, typically increases in numbers. Exercise makes fit bugs produce more antioxidants, more healthy chemicals, and we benefit. Fit people have fit gut bugs.

You will hear a lot more of this in the future as it is a rapidly developing field. Your gut bugs may influence performance and the right bugs may help you to run faster. The additional antioxidants produced by good bugs may be the key or the healthy chemicals such as free fatty acids also play a role by interacting positively with muscles. Personalized sport nutrition is developing to include targeting of gut bugs, particularly now in elite athletes.

Environment

The place where you live is a major determinant of the composition of your gut bugs. The features of gut microbiota are unique to different locations and lifestyles. Gut bugs vary depending on whether you live in high- or low-income countries and whether you live in industrialized or traditional rural communities. City dwellers have different gut bugs than those people living in rural environments.

Even an apparently healthy Western gut has a poor range of microbial diversity compared to traditional cultures. People living in American cities, have less diverse bugs, with species loss compared to those living in traditional rural communities in South America and Africa.[88] Asians who emigrate to the US develop rapid loss of diversity of their gut bugs. The longer immigrants stay in the US, the more their gut bugs approach the US type.[89] Traditional rural populations have higher bug diversity and novel bugs, compared to urbanized Western gut microbiota. As countries prosper, there is loss of gut bug diversity.

We share many of the gut bugs with the people that live with us. It doesn't matter if you are genetically related or not, the household shares its gut bugs. Living with someone, rather than living alone, means it is more likely that you have lots of diverse gut bugs. And furthermore, if you have a close relationship with that person, you have an even larger diversity of gut bugs. Pets bring something to the party also; we share our skin bugs with our four-legged friends.

We don't fully understand the reasons for the variations of our gut bugs from country to country and person to person. It may be a complex interplay of our food, water, lifestyle and genes. It is difficult to give a normal reference range for our gut bugs, because of these differences.[90]

Fasting

You may be worried that fasting will harm your gut bugs. I have a close mental relationship with my gut bugs, and I don't like to think of them starving. I was pretty relieved to find, that on the contrary, fasting allows regeneration and clearing out of the dead wood. Fasting is a natural state in the animal kingdom, hibernation being an extreme example. Animals too have gut microbiota. During hibernation, the gut bugs of squirrels change, survive and thrive on awakening.[91] In two weeks, there is a robust return to production of healthy short chain fatty acids, essential for health and produced by the gut bugs. Who knew that gut bugs hibernated?

In humans, intermittent fasting has been shown to increase diversity of gut bugs.[92] Good bugs, such as Akkermansia increase in number from fasting like they do from exercise.[93] Fasting has been shown to have significant benefits in the laboratory. It increases the ratio of good to bad bugs, increases production of healthy short chain fatty acids and is associated with reduced insulin sensitivity.[94] Increased levels of serotonin and other chemicals required for brain health and happiness, have been demonstrated with intermittent fasting, which may be due to the effect on our gut bugs.[95]

Humans have fasted for millions of years and gut bugs, evolving with us, are accustomed to periods of fasting. Fasting was part of our lives, as food supply was often irregular. Periods of fasting are good for both us and our gut bugs. We don't do well on 4-6 meals and snacks a day and our gut bugs don't either.[96,97]

WHO HAS GOOD BUGS?

We live in a fragile world which has survived five mass extinctions over 500 million years, wiping out 99% of species. We are now seeing catastrophic plant and animal extinctions, but as yet, the loss does not represent a mass extinction. A rich diversity of gut bugs is seen in people with traditional lifestyles. This rich diversity of the gut is not seen in the modern gut in high-income countries. Some experts believe that the present wave of extinction is now affecting our gut bugs.

The Hadza people have gut bugs that probably more reflects our ancestral bugs more closely than any other peoples. Their gut bugs are entirely unique, highly diverse, with combinations not seen elsewhere. Many of the bugs are unknown to us and have never been seen before. The Hadza people have good bugs. They do not suffer from modern diseases, such as hypertension, metabolic syndrome, diabetes or cancer, which may be related to their healthy gut bugs.

Not so long ago, the national rugby teams drank, made merry and were overweight. That is no longer the case. These men are supreme athletes, lean and fit. The Irish rugby team have good gut bugs. They have a richly diverse colony with good proportions of good bugs and no nasty ones. Exercise, fitness, diet and the fine sport of Rugby, all contribute to their healthy guts.

HOW DO I LOOK AFTER MY GUT BUGS?

The biggest win is to feed your gut microbiota. If you feed them properly, the bugs themselves will feed other bugs, which in turn will create a good, diverse colony of gut bugs. Fasting, exercise, a good sleep pattern and being part of nature will help your gut bugs. Avoid antibiotics, unless you are seriously ill and there are no safe alternatives. The key is in the name. Biotic is a living thing, anti is against, so an antibiotic is a drug that is against living things.

Prebiotics are foodstuffs that provide food, in the form of fiber, to your gut microbiota. Prebiotics help good bacteria to grow. Prebiotics are present in fiber rich foods such as vegetables, wholegrains, fruits, seeds and nuts. And we know that people with high fiber diets have fewer diseases and live longer. Prebiotics in foods directly influence the gut bugs in a positive way. You need to eat lots of prebiotics. To do this, you should eat plants and eat lots of different plants.

Probiotics are foodstuffs which contain live bugs, teaming with cultures of good bacteria. They are fermented foods, which have been shown to have several beneficial effects on health and benefit to the gut bugs. Fermented foods include bioactive yogurts, kefir, sauerkraut tempeh, miso, kombucha, pickles and fermented vegetables. Cheeses made from raw milk are also good probiotic food, teaming with live bacterial cultures.

The Food and Drug Administration is tasked with protecting the American population. In a major "safety advance" in 2014, they banned cheeses made from raw or unpasteurized milk. Now you know why your cheese plate in America lacks cheeses such as Comte, Brie, Roquefort and some Cheddar. There are lots of other live cheeses; just look for "raw or unpasteurized milk' on the label. We always have Comte in our house. There is no agreement whether probiotics in food are better than probiotics in supplements, but Paul and I are sticking to natural food sources. This concurs with the views of many others.[98]

At the start of our food discovery journey, we introduced fermented vegetables to our diet. We eat a lot of salads and thought pickled red cabbage and sauerkraut were an easy win. Paul wasn't so pleased, but he munched his way through the cabbage, thinking of all the happy gut bugs. About a year later, we realized that vegetables pickled in vinegar do not have live bacterial cultures, only vegetables pickled in salt and water have live bacterial cultures. Vinegar is a great food, but not in this instance. Our experiment had been entirely in vain. Check labels and ingredients carefully, or better still, ferment your own vegetables.

Kefir is fermented milk teeming with lots of good bugs. Called "grains of the prophet", it has been drunk for over four thousand years, and we still talk of the lumps of live bacteria as "grains". For the sake of clarity, these have no relationship with grains from grasses. Kefir has long been considered to have magical properties. The kefir grains were secretly passed from generation to generation, amongst the people of the Caucasus mountains. The grains were so valuable that they were considered to part of a family's wealth. Kefir is now widely available but is very easy to make yourself. You need a starter culture, which will live in perpetuity.

But introducing kefir to your diet may be an interesting experiment. Some years ago, we were in Slovenia, endurance swimming in the mountain lakes. It is a glorious part of the world, and we journeyed into the Alps to find ourselves alone in spectacular clear lakes, with only the fish for company. Slovenia had a peaceful feel and the people lead simple agrarian lives. The shops reflected this, and I found some kefir, something I had wanted to try for some time, but had not been able to source. Greedily drinking my kefir, I was very pleased with the new additions to my gut bugs. Paul watched with mounting suspicion. Early the next morning, I headed off as usual for a 10 km run around lake Bohinj. At 6 km in, all my metrics went pear-shaped, my heart rate was up, my pace slowed, and then with more than a degree of urgency, I headed for the bushes. Armageddon had occurred in my gut, with a massive punch up between the new guys and the old brigade. And it has to be said with little concern for their caring host. It was the only time in my life I had produced a perfect replica cowpat. You have been warned. It only happens once, then peace breaks out.

FREQUENTLY ASKED QUESTIONS

What does a healthy gut microbiota do?

It helps to protect you and maintain your immune system. It helps to digest your food and make vitamins. It helps your brain health by making hormone like messengers. It produces a host of chemicals, which contribute to your overall functioning and well-being.

What makes a healthy gut microbiota?

A healthy microbiota has lots of different organisms and species. A rich and highly diverse collection is a good indicator of a healthy microbiota. There is a preponderance of good bugs, a low number of bad bugs and very low numbers of dangerous bugs.

What is the quickest win to improve my gut bugs?

You should eat different sources of fiber from a range of diverse foods. The greater the number of varied plant foods, the better. Your diet would look like this: lots of vegetables, legumes, beans, wholegrains, seeds, nuts and fruit, in addition to protein and fats. You should avoid processed foods, particularly those with high sugar content such as biscuits, cakes, white bread, donut, fruit juices, white pasta, smoothies, sodas, pies, ice-cream, readymade sauces, and "healthy" low-fat snacks. These foods feed your bad bugs. Diet sodas should be avoided as artificial sweeteners have been shown in animal studies to disrupt gut bugs. If you do this, your good bugs will thrive, and your bad bugs will suffer and decline. Your gut bugs will change rapidly within a few days. Beneficial effects on your body will take a bit longer to become apparent. Stick with it.

Should I eat prebiotics?

Yes. Prebiotics refers to food containing fiber, which promotes the growth of good bugs. Prebiotics are critical for health. Eat fiber from diverse foods sources, which will promote the growth of a variety of good bugs. Prebiotics are the foods and fertilizer for your gut bugs.

Should I eat probiotics?

Yes. Probiotics are foods which contains live bacterial cultures. Probiotics add new species to your gut bugs. Diversity of your gut bugs is one of the markers of a healthy gut microbiota. Probiotics include yogurt, kefir, pickles, miso, kombucha, tempeh, kimchi and fermented vegetables, such as sauerkraut. Probiotics are the new seeds of your new gut "cottage garden". Make sure that you check the labels, looking for 'live cultures'. When you consider your gut bugs to be a cottage garden, it helps you to look after them. Watering and feeding them but keeping away the pesticides.

What else can I do?

Lifestyle affects your gut bugs. Look at different aspects of your life, such as fasting, exercise, sleep, time spent outdoors and socializing.

How can I get Christensenella into my gut?

Christensenella is a highly desirable component of the gut bugs. This is a bug that you really want to have. People who live to over 100, are particularly healthy, and they have a relative abundance of Christensenella. There is current work looking at commercializing this bug and developing a Christensenella drug candidate. It's not available now but may be available in the future. But you don't need supplements and you don't need pills; look after your gut bugs, eat a diverse range of foods and plants, and it will flourish.

Will my gut microbiota improve if I look after it?

Yes. If you alter your diet and lifestyle, your gut microbiota will change. You can restore diversity. You can restore the proportions of good to bad bugs and you will then reap the rewards.

What does the future hold for good bug assessments?

You will have your gut bugs analyzed on a regular basis. Management of conditions will include treatment of your gut bugs. Your medical treatment, your food and fasting regimes will be personalized for you on the basis of your gut bugs. Gut bugs will play a big part of all our lives.

CHAPTER WHISPERINGS

- Our bodies exist in harmony with 39 trillion of bugs in our gut

- Our health and well-being are dependent on our gut bugs

- Our gut bugs perform many functions that we humans are unable to do

- Our gut bugs protect us, feed us, supply chemicals that control our moods, appetite and metabolism

- Traditional cultures have a more diverse and healthier gut microbiota than Western cultures

- In health, the relationship between our gut bugs and ourselves is mutually beneficial

- Dysbiosis, where there is a perturbation of the composition of the gut bugs is associated with many modern conditions such as obesity, hypertension, diabetes and cancer

- Maintaining healthy gut bugs is critical for wellness

- A healthy diverse diet with plenty of fiber, exercise, sleep, fasting, environment, probiotics and socialization all help to support healthy gut bugs

- You could think of your gut microbiota as a beautiful and varied cottage garden. Feed and nurture, it well, and it will grow and reward you with good health

CHAPTER 11

UNDERSTANDING YOUR OWN FAT

*"The lunches of fifty-seven years had caused his chest to slip down into the mez-
zanine floor"*

P.G. Wodehouse

INTRODUCTION

It is important to know that our body fat is spiraling up or spiraling down;
it's never in a steady state. Here we are dealing not with the fat we eat, but
with our own stored body fat, the good the bad and the ugly. Our body fat
includes;

Sub-cutaneous fat; the pinch an inch variety (as we saw in figure 2.1); this
helps to keep us warm and giggles around when we move. It's on our back,
our legs, in fact all over the body. Generally, women have more of it than
men. It is an effective insulator and protective layer not only in us, but in
marine animals such as seals and whales. This is not the dangerous sort of
fat and in moderation has some health advantages

- Intramuscular fat; the fat within our muscles, which is a normal part of
  our fat stores

- Liver fat; the most active part of the fat stores. This fat is turned into
  sugar, when our glycogen stores are low. It is also used to make ketone
  bodies when we are fasting

- Orbital fat; like other fats provide physical protection to our organs, in
  this case the eyes. People can get into a terrible mess with the balance
  between the eyes, when this fat is damaged or removed

- Cell walls; every cell has fat in the form of lipoproteins in the cell wall

- Neurological fat; 60% of our brain and neurological tissues are fat. Yes, I did say that! Dietary fats, in the form of omega-3s are required for good fetal brain development, and may also be protective against many other neurological diseases, including dementia[7,99]

- Hormones; many are made from fats

- Fat cells; also release their own hormones

- Vitamin transport; fat soluble vitamins A, D, E and K require fat for absorption from the gut

- Visceral fat; the bad boy

We know that most dietary fats are essential to our well-being. Here we see that body fat is also intrinsic to our survival.

VISCERAL FAT

Visceral fat is the real bad boy of fat, and present in over 80% of obese people. It is also present in over 80% of people in the USA that are not traditionally fat; these we call metabolically fat.[100] This was first recognized as metabolically obese normal weight (MONW), 29 years ago.[101] These people range from normal weight to overweight, but their scans and bloods are abnormal; they too go on to get metabolic syndrome and the associated medical problems listed below. In this group we know as BMI increases, so do the risks of metabolic problems and illnesses.[102] This is common in south Indians and Asians. In America, it is estimated that an eye watering 88% of all US adults have abnormal blood tests and scans, which leads to metabolic syndrome.[103] Metabolic syndrome means big trouble down the road. Big risk factors for MONW are lack of exercise, increasing weight and high alcohol consumption, the consumption of refined and super-refined carbohydrates and high frequency meals.[104] This includes soda drinks and low-fat foods, both laced with high fructose corn syrup.

Overweight people aged over 65, with a BMI in the range 27-29 have a reduced risk of death from all causes. In this group weight loss is inadvisable on BMI alone, unless they have visceral fat and metabolic risks. At younger ages, we know obesity is unstable and risks progressing to metabolic syndrome, so weight loss is recommended.[104]

Visceral fat produces so many hormones that it is considered an organ in its own right. We have created in our bellies a hormone producing monster. And bad hormones too, 20 of which are identified. We are still far from knowing all their effects on us. I'll be willing to wager a bet that no great new stories will emerge from this group of hormones. Hormones produced are leptin, adinopectin, ADMTS-1, chemerin, resistin, and the list goes on; what a hormonal hellfire soup our visceral fat is!

So, we know that visceral fat is the baddy and causes metabolic syndrome. Everyone should differentiate harmful visceral fat, from friendly subcutaneous fat. People with a BMI above normal, must watch for progression to visceral fat. In the US 36.2% of the population are obese. That is 119 million people of whom 80% will have visceral fat and metabolic syndrome. Worryingly, 80% of all adults, fat or thin, in the US have at least one abnormal metabolic marker of metabolic syndrome. That amounts to 167 million people. That is an unmitigated disaster of world war proportions.

METABOLIC SYNDROME

Metabolic syndrome is a combination of high blood pressure, abnormal cholesterol, insulin resistance and increased abdominal girth. This ranges from the grossly obese, to a stick thin individual with a tiny pot-belly, as is often seen in South Indian men. The international definition is;

- Waist >37 inches (>94 cm in men) or >31 inches (>80 cm in women) along with the presence of two or more of the following:

- Blood glucose greater than 5.6 mmol/L (100 mg/dl) or diagnosed diabetes

- HDL cholesterol 1.0 mmol/L (40 mg/dl) in men, <1.3 mmol/L (50 mg/dl) in women or drug treatment for low HDL

- Blood triglycerides >1.7 mmol/L (150 mg/dl) or drug treatment for elevated triglycerides

- Blood pressure >130/85 mmHg or drug treatment for hypertension

Unchecked metabolic syndrome is associated with just about every non-communicable disease known to man. Cancer of the prostate, breast, pancreas and others, type 2 diabetes, high blood pressure, heart disease, strokes, gout, psychological problems, neurological diseases, renal problems, birth obesity, childhood obesity, infertility in women, changed menstrual cycles, hypogonadism, infertility, Polycystic ovarian syndrome, erectile dysfunction, lichen planus, SLE, psoriasis, acanthosis nigrans, inflammation, fat cell inflammation with changed CRP, IL-1, IL-6, adinopectin and leptin resistance, joint problems, rheumatoid arthritis, oxidative stress, leaky bowel, reduced gut microbiota diversity, small bowel microbial overgrowth, sleep apnea, schizophrenia, tiredness, non-alcoholic fatty liver disease, road traffic accidents, Polycystic ovarian syndrome, thyroid dysfunction, hormonal problems, insulin resistance, diabetes, visual dysfunction, cataracts, macular degeneration, diabetic eye disease and blindness, retina artery occlusion, retinal vein occlusion, lower lid entropion; the list goes on and on.[105,106,107] Primary gout in normal weight people is associated with metabolic syndrome.[105] Every extra inch around your waste from visceral fat increases your cardiovascular risks by 5%.[108,109,110,111]

And, as we have seen, this is not only a personal problem, but a societal problem too. Metabolic syndrome will eventually overwhelm our healthcare systems. Governments and the medical profession need to wake up to this crisis. We cannot treat our way out of metabolic syndrome; it has to be prevention, early detection and reversal. Our leaders will need to be tough enough to take on the bleating liberals and libertarians.

CAUSES OF METABOLIC SYNDROME

The question is a simple one that deserves a simple answer. This list explains with clarity, what causes metabolic syndrome. With the same certainty the corollary is true; remove these causes from your life and your metabolic syndrome disappears. The diet-whisperer plan will guide you through this. The culprits are;

- Super-refined carbohydrates

- Refined carbohydrates

- High meal frequency

- Snacking

- Fructose and high fructose corn syrup, HFCS45 and HFCS55

- Soda drinks

- Low-fat foods laced with HFCS

- High cortisol and chronic stress

- Obesity, in the form of visceral fat

- Lack of exercise

- Diet high omega-6 to omega-3 ratio

- Smoking

EARLY SIGNS OF METABOLIC SYNDROME

For early detection, we need to be able to determine who has visceral fat and quantify it. Then remeasure it after the necessary lifestyle changes have taken place. The gold standard test is a CT scan, but these are expensive and give you a fair wallop of radiation, making it a non-starter for repeated testing in people who want to look after their health. The next best test is a DEXA scan, which is cheaper, correlates well with the CT scan and is 0.003 the radiation exposure, so is suitable for repeated measurements of visceral fat. Ultra-sound in good hands is also effective.

Then there is a whole raft of anthropometric tests; easily done measurements at home. These include thigh to waist ratios, height to waist ratio, and a whole host of others. Your BMI can be calculated on our website, using height and weight as the two variables. It was originally called the Quetelet index after its Belgian inventor Adolphe Quetelet in the 19th century as a measurement of body fat. A normal value for BMI is 18.5 to 24.9, underweight is less than 18.5, overweight is 25.0 to 29.9 and obesity is classified as a BMI over 30.

BMI is an assessment of overall fat content, and we have seen that his correlates poorly with visceral fat; its accuracy is also affected by age, ethnicity, sex and muscle mass, and it correlates poorly with the risk of metabolic syndrome.

But beware, a high BMI without metabolic syndrome indicates an increased risk of type II diabetes.[112] A high BMI is associated with increased death from all causes.[110] A low BMI in smokers confers no protection.[111]

The two most popular home tests are abdominal circumference and hip-to-waist ratio. You simply divide the circumference of your waist at the level of your belly button, by the circumference of your hips at the widest point. If you can feel the top of your pelvic bone on either side above your hips, that is the ideal height for a waist measurement keeping the tape at that level all the way around your tummy. The WHO recommends for women a ratio of less than 0.85 and men 0.90. People with a normal BMI, who have a high hip-to-waist ratio, doubles the risk of cardiovascular disease.[108,109]

A term you may come across is the android : gynoid ratio, which is a DEXA scan ratio of fat levels between the visceral fat and subcutaneous fat. In other words, a DEXA scan version of the hip to waist ratio. A high ratio in children and adolescents is associated with insulin resistance and indicates a poorer health in the future for those children.[113] They will have a life plagued by chronic diseases and an earlier death. We should be protecting our children. If this is not a priority of government then why not?

Any of these simple tests that give abnormal readings should warrant a further investigation of your visceral fat by DEXA scan and blood tests from your doctor to see if you have metabolic syndrome, pre-diabetes or diabetes. No matter what age you are, your life is in your hands. Seize the moment.

MEN AND WOMEN'S FAT

Women naturally have more fat than men. Normal fat percentage of body weight is 18-25% in men increasing with age, and in women 21-35%. Obesity is associated with fat >25% in men and >32% in women. In athletes, body fat may be as low as 10% (7-13) in men and 17% (14-20) in women. Your body fat and other measurements can be calculated at www.diet-whisperer.com.

FAT CELLS; SIZE, AGE AND LEPTIN

Fat cells are called adipocytes. When our hormone insulin causes fat to be laid down, it does so in fatty tissues in two ways. Firstly, in adults more fat, in the form of triglyceride, is stuffed into each fat cell, making them bigger. The number of these fat cells remains remarkably constant throughout adulthood. And secondly, only in our teenage years are we able to lay down more fat cells.

So, when adults get fatter, they do so within the fat cells they already own. But when teenagers get fat, they do the same, but additionally lay down more fat cells. Adolescent obesity results in an increased number of fat cells for life. This is deeply shocking. We are setting our kids up to fail.

In adulthood, we keep a remarkably constant number of fat cells, around 15 billion.[8] Turnover is remarkably low, with about 10% dying and being replaced every year, and stored triglycerides on average hanging around inside the cells for about 2 years. With certainty, big pharma is looking at the chemical inhibition of the "new fat cells" produced as part of this natural turnover, as a site for new drugs.[114] This utopian panacea that we can eat what we want, then shed it with a pill is not only fool's gold, but it will not happen. Those that want this, probably also want eternal life; which misses the very essence of life itself.

Leptin is our satiety hormone; it tells us we're satisfied and full. It is produced by fat cells and sends a message to our brain to stop eating. My late father Derick taught me that the right time to leave a party is just before you want to. So, apologies to all my friends on the occasions I've ignored his sage advice and stayed for just one last drink! Similarly, the Japanese say, "stop eating before you're full". Good strong advice from a country ranking 6th from bottom in the world rankings for obesity at 4.3% of the population; they share an average body mass index of 22.60 and share some of the longest life expectancy on earth. Okinawa, in Japan, one of the world's Blue Zones, is an example of a place where people do not have metabolic syndrome. These Blue Zones will be discussed in the wellness chapter.

There is a bit more to this aspect of leptin. You see leptin release, tells us we've had enough and is a strong driver to go all Japanese at mealtime. And, leptin release is greatest from fat cells that are few in number and big. Leptin release is lowest from fat cells that are large in number and small; just how they are in an overweight teenager. More problems trying to lose weight later in life and another reason to prevent obesity in the young.

FAT AS AN ENERGY STORE

Let us consider one aspect of our fat stores; energy. Fat provides us with energy to burn. Every second we live, breath and our heart still beats, we require energy. So yes, vegging out in front of the TV burns about 2000 calories per day in your average teenage Kevin. The number of calories we burn each day is known as our basal metabolic rate (BMR). If you happen to have a Kevin vegging on your sofa, feel free to cover this section with indelible marker pen. By walking 1-mile Kevin would burn about 100 calories. And Kevin knows that lying on the couch watching The Grand Tour, will burn 83 calories per hour. So why bother with the walk; Kevin has a point. Calories in versus out is a nonsense I shall debunk later. Kevin knows that his favorite can of soda will give him 150 calories. So, if he has a soda every few hours, he'll be pretty much OK; from the calorie argument at least. And roughly, his maths is OK, but if only life was that simple. The soda has the equivalent of something like 13 sugar cubes.

When we stoke the fire on a steam engine we do so with coal. Why, because it is a fantastically energy dense black glossy rock called anthracite. It was laid down and compressed from dead plants in swamp lands in the carboniferous period some 300 million years ago. It is more than fifty percent carbon, which is why Greta Thunberg hates it, and why the Chinese electricity generators love it. Its energy density is 7 calories per gram (cal/g). As a comparison gasoline is 10 cal/g, and natural gas 13cal/g. How does that compare with our body's fuels? Well, carbohydrates are 4 cal/g, proteins 4 cal/g and, wait for it, fat is 9 cal/g. So fat, as we can see is our miracle store of energy. I shall teach you how to utilize your own fat to your advantage; quite the opposite to fearing its calorie density as a food.

An 80 kg man and 50 kg women have a daily calorie burn, or BMR of 1500 cal/day and 1200 cal/day respectively, at the age of fifty. This reduces by roughly 2% per decade. BMR does not differentiate between fat and muscular build types, and it has its limitations because BMR makes no assessment of activity. When we talk of Total Energy Expenditure (TEE) we can multiply the BMR by factors depending on activities of individuals for example light activity (1.53), moderate (1.76) or vigorous (2.25). These would equate to office worker, factory worker and agricultural worker. In exercise terms, these factors would equate to walking for less that 1 hour, running for 1 hour, running faster for over 1 hour respectively. We have a calculator for you on the website to play with. So, sorry Kevin has five problems;

- Activity does change BMR

- Exercise, even walking is really beneficial for your health

- Calorie counting doesn't work, and I'll debunk this in diet mythology

- Kevin has, or will have, Soda Drink Syndrome (SDS)

- Kevin is already on the bus route to metabolic syndrome

DODGING BULLETS

Dodging bullets is our metaphor, for getting the balance right. As we progress through life, we have a stream of bullets, fired from afar and flying towards us. At the diet-whisperer we're far from perfect. Our philosophy is not to rid ourselves of all risk, but to allow us to eat well, drink, be sociable, laugh a lot, be mentally and physically well, and enjoy life free of all those inflammatory diseases. We want the bullets to be fewer, and get the balance right, so we can avoid as many flesh wounds as possible. Diet-whispering is about living life to the full, but realistically and as healthily as possible.

CHAPTER WHISPERINGS

- Visceral fat is known as belly fat and is the dangerous fat we cannot see or feel
- Visceral fat is metabolically active and dangerous long term
- Fat is an essential food
- Differentiating the two types of fat is important for us to know
- We have seen that subcutaneous fat is not a problem per se
- The brain is 60% fat
- Metabolic syndrome has been defined
- BMI can be easily calculated but has limitations for race and build type
- Other anthropometric tests exist that are better measure of visceral fat
- Visceral fat can occur in otherwise thin individuals
- Women have more total body fat than men
- Fat is an almost infinite store of energy and is energy dense
- Visceral fat is caused by refined carbohydrates in the diet
- BMR can be calculated to see our daily calorific needs and modified for activity levels
- The diet-whisperer plan will put you in control for quick health benefits

CHAPTER 12

BODY SHAPE AND RATIO D'OR

"Take Care of your body. It's the only place you have to live."

Jim Rohn

INTRODUCTION

I get asked these a lot. Blokes, how do I get rid of my fat face, love handles and belly? And girls, how do I lose weight off my bum, but not my boobs? The answer to these questions is always the same; you can't shape your fat. Full stop. No pills, no specific exercises will "target" your fat loss. It comes off where and when it wants. The good news is that your visceral fat will be attacked first, with some quick metabolic gains to boot. Quick gains and feeling better.

EXERCISE

We should all exercise for our mental and physical health. Not for fat loss. Let me expand on this concept. In 2019, Monique did her first full 140.6 Ironman triathlon, in Vitoria-Gastiez, Spain. And a beautiful place too, where the locals made us very welcome. At 59 years of age, she trained 17 hours per week. The full Ironman is an open water swim of 3.8 km (c. 2.4 miles) followed by a 190 km (c. 118 mi miles) cycle and then a full marathon of 42.2 km (c. 26 miles). All at a temperature in the high 30's Celsius. After a half Ironman the previous year, she trained for one year, covering a total distance of 4,457 kilometers, with an altitude gain the equivalent to climbing Mount Everest three times over. Her total training over twelve months was 349 hours! Some achievement, for which she has my, and I suspect your, utmost respect. And here's the rub! She didn't lose

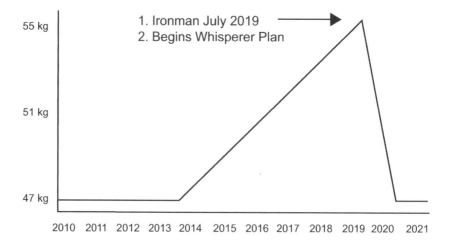

Figure 12.1. Monique's weight over 8 years of triathlon training with regular exercise and very little alcohol. The triathlon distances increased from sprint triathlon to olympic then half and full ironman. Over the 8 years the training and distances increased, but so did the weight, inspite of an excellent diet.

a single pound in the whole year. From the chart you can see her weight gain over 8 years of triathlon (figure 12.1). This was suddenly punctuated by a serious skiing accident on the Klein Matterhorn, in which she badly ruptured her right knee ligaments. Yes, there was a muscle component, but that was not the whole story. She eats an uber sensible diet and almost drank no alcohol for that whole year. Her personal desires, like many women, are less upper arm fat, less belly fat, and a slimmer waist. And lastly, to achieve the golden ratio.

MUSCLE

Resistance training, or weight training, should be part of everyone's routine beyond the age of thirty. The reason for this is that after the age of 30 we start to naturally lose our muscles. And, there is never a time when it's too late to start building and training your muscles. Maybe that extra muscle strength will save you from a fall when you're 93. And you'll say thanks to the diet-whisperer. Falls in older people are associated with the same risk as death as a diagnosis of cancer; yep, they're bad news. And why do the elderly fall? The reasons are poor muscle strength, and loss of balance, which again can be trained for on a daily basis. That's good solid wisdom to carry with you throughout life. The speed at which you walk, and the time that you can balance on one leg with your eyes closed, both correlate with your life expectancy. And both can be trained.

So, for muscle growth you can "target" which muscle to grow. Unlike fat, muscle can be sculpted. Muscle is of two general types, cardiac and skeletal, and they're very similar but work on very different fuels. Also, you'll be glad that cardiac muscle is very much automatic and run by the autonomic nervous system. Your skeletal muscle is controlled consciously by your motor nervous system connecting your brain to each muscle. When humans sleep, unlike many animals, we lose muscle tone, which is why we don't sleep in trees! An exception is when I bang your knee with a patella hammer, or you inadvertently put your hand on the hot kettle. These involuntary reflexes are relays around the spine and based on the good concept that harm can come to you before your brain knows it. Particularly if you've been out at the pub. They cut out the thinking bit.

There are three types of skeletal muscle fibers. The first type I is called a slow-twitch (ST) fiber which you use for walking or jogging. The second is a fast-twitch (FT), which comes in two varieties, FT-I and FT-II.

If you want endurance, you train your slow twitch fibers, and these do not increase in size with training. You train them by respecting the 80-20 rule.[115] That is slow and long for 80% of the time and high intensity interval training (HIIT) for 20%. If you believe anyone, even doctors telling you there is a shortcut to endurance fitness by increasing your HIIT you must not believe them.[116]

If you want to change your shape, you can achieve this with overall fat loss and targeted muscle growth. And no-one will be impressed if your beautifully sculpted muscles lie under a blanket of fat. Remember seals are very muscular creatures. Most people have 6-packs, it's just that they're covered in seal blubber!

Each muscle has a mixture of these three types of fiber. Overall humans are 60% fast-twitch and 40% slow-twitch. There are genetic variations and elite distance runners are born with a higher proportion of slow twitch, and Usain Bolt we could safely bet, has a higher proportion of fast twitch fibers. However, it should be noted that whilst we cannot change the ratio of fibers we're born with, we can train one type of fiber to work a little more like another type. As well as the propensity of fiber type, the volume of our muscle is an inherited variable. And no matter how good our genes are at gifting us the right amount and types of muscle fibers, champions still need to put the work in to become champions. The corollary to this is that no matter how hard one trains, one has a gene encoded upper limit. In other words, no matter how hard Usain Bolt trains he could never become a champion marathon runner. Another important message here is that at any age, you can get fitter and stronger and build muscle.

And whilst we're talking muscle fiber types and composition, the fastest animal on earth the cheetah, has 75% fast-twitch fibers. If you want to escape a cheetah, sitting in his Baobab tree, then firstly run like hell in the opposite direction and secondly don't stop. As the old adage goes, you don't need to outrun the predator, just the guy next to you. The cheetah is only in contact with the ground for 5 seconds over 100 meters, using his tail as a rudder and reaching 75 mph (c. 120 km/h). Your human advantage is that of endurance. A cheetah will stop after 500 meters, fast twitch fibers drained of all their fuel, and he will lope back to his Baobab, as the energy slowly returns to his fast twitch fibers. Our anthropogenic resilience is due to our roughly equal measure of sprinting and endurance. The reason you're alive and reading this is because of the endurance ability of your ancestors to hunt and evade.

Slow-twitch fibers do not expand during training, which is why cycling supremo Sir Bradley Wiggins, has such successful yet slender legs. And Sir Bradley's training would have induced many new mitochondria (our cellular power stations) into his slow twitch fibers. Slow twitch fibers use oxygen in the mitochondria as a catalyst for fueling. Think middle through long distance to ultra-marathon runners and cyclists.

Fast-twitch fibers do expand through weight training. And, if looking like Popeye is your thing, then resistance training is for you. If you target the FT-I fibers, you'll be doing 70-80% the maximum you can lift once (MaxR1) for 10-20 repetitions (reps) for 3-6 sets. FT-I fibers are particularly good for power and sprinting and team sports like rugby and football. Think 400 metres. They have moderate numbers of mitochondria but utilize mainly non-oxygen (anaerobic) cell-based fuels for short burst of energy, then fatigue quickly. The FT-I fibers can expand by 25%, thus shaping your physique.

But if you really want that sculpted look, here's a great tip; go for your FT-II fibers. These are used by power lifters. They have low blood and oxygen supply and fewer mitochondria, so fatigue quickly. But they can grow by a massive 100%. Think here very explosive bursts over 30-100 meters. Resistance training would require lifting to failure, and lower reps at 90-95% of your MaxR1.

So, in terms of targeting, it is possible to favor one set of muscles to build, in whichever way you want. Take for example a Tour de France cyclist, like Sir Bradley. If you are going to win the Tour overall, known as the GC, you will need to target your muscles in training. The race ahead is 2175 miles (c. 3,500 km) over twenty stages and the important bit, is that the course will take you up 66,000 feet (c. 20,000 m) of elevation. You will average 25mph (c. 40 km/h) and burn 125,000 kcal. Those are big numbers.

Training must focus on the right muscles, and the right muscle fibers. And, as anyone who has done long cycle climbs knows, the lighter the bike, the better. But the biggest weight saving is on the rider himself. So, target the muscles; get the strongest legs and the weakest arms. Imagine, being able to build very strong endurance resistant legs, but getting rid of the arm muscle that then in turn does not have to be carried as excess baggage. And if the core of the body is strong, the arms can be even thinner and have even less muscle.

How to do this is easy in theory, but in practice requires total dedication in training. Muscles when being trained get damaged. They are made from protein, and extra protein in the diet is required to rebuild muscle over the following week. Dietary protein is then utilized by the body to rebuild the damaged muscle. Top teams spend both time and energy assessing the exact dietary mix of carbs to refuel and store as glycogen, and protein to repair the muscle and healthy fats to provide nutrition. But, if you exercise the legs and not the arms and restrict dietary protein, then you can "steal" new leg protein by breaking down the protein in the arms. Ever wondered why pro cyclists look like they do? Now you know.

YOU CAN'T OUTRUN YOUR KITCHEN

I have my old theater sister Carrie to thank for teaching me this saying. The only people who can are supreme athletes at the top of their game; those who can exercise for 6-8 hours per day. The elite cyclists along with cross-country skiers and ultramarathon runners, are an exception to the rule that you can't outrun your kitchen. These amazing people can. In fact, in Dean Karnazes' enthralling book "The Confessions of a Midnight Runner" he describes ordering a takeout pizza at night with coffee which he balances on his forearm and eats as he runs.[117] But remember unless you're one of these extraordinary folks, you won't outrun a bad diet! Also, important to remember is that when you do run more and do more cardio, if your diet is restricted, your body's hormones will turn down your metabolism, in a race of diet versus metabolism. And the important point is that your hormones will always win; they will beat you every time. If not at month one, month two or even month twelve, you'll lose. Exercise because you like it. Exercise to live longer, to feel better and be fitter and stronger. But do not ever exercise to lose weight. It's frustrating and in the battle with your hormones, you will lose. So, yes for absolutely definitely sure you should exercise, but not for weight loss. Let diet-whispering do that bit for you. Putting you in control of how you look and feel, for the short term and forever.

FAT SHAPING

So, we can see that it is very possible to target and shape certain muscles, through different exercises and dietary manipulation. So, what about fat? Sorry, but the truth is you cannot target fat loss from targeted dieting nor targeted exercising. You've seen the adverts for "no more upper arm fat" on this pill, or that exercise etc. It doesn't work; it's a con.

Of course, I can tell you that if you are a 40-year-old woman and you want to get rid of the flabby arms, first you have to reduce your overall body fat content. It will come off everywhere at the same time. And yes, your boobs will get smaller too.

When you lose weight through hormone realignment, you can then burn off the arm fat, along with everything else. Then you can build your triceps, biceps and deltoids . This will make your arms and shoulders more defined.

LEG CELLULITE

And here is the greatest home truth for women. Fat is metabolically inert, and has little blood flow, hence cellulite, or those dimples along the upper arms and thighs. To rid yourself of cellulite, you will need to increase the vascularity of your fat. Fat vascularization occurs with aerobic endurance sports, such as running. We have seen dramatic disappearance of leg cellulite with people who have taken up long distance running.

This also indicates an improved metabolic state with regard to blood glucose control and changes in chemicals called FOXO proteins.[118] So new blood vessels growing into your fat is not only gets rid of cellulite but is metabolically beneficial too. There you have it. For women the cost of this book may well be worth that simple piece of knowledge. Running shoes on and go longer!

THE GOLDEN RATIO

This is one of nature's most beautiful stories. The Fibonacci sequence is the sequence of numbers that go 1,1,2,3,5,8,13,21,34,55 etc. See if you can spot the sequence. The answer is a basic mathematical sequence; add any number to the previous number, to get the following number. And where this gets interesting is if we divide any larger number by the preceding number, we get 13/8 = 1.625; 21/13=1.615; 55/34 = 1.618. And as we go on, we get closer and closer to 1.162, but never reach it. So, the divided Fibonacci numbers "tend" to 1.62, but never reach it.

In nature 1.618 is the Golden ratio. The Golden Ratio is simply everywhere in nature, from the length of branches on a tree, to the hand to forearm ratio in humans, and the ratios found inside cells and shells. And, humans have used this ratio for perfect house and window proportions, the Parthenon as well as many other architectural delights. It's used in art and advertising to please you and suck you in. Even da Vinci's Mona Lisa. The Golden Ratio, also known by the Greek letter phi.

When a woman looks at a man from the back she instinctively, yet subconsciously calculates his shoulder to waist ratio. In the ideal lean man, like Michelangelo's David, this perfect and pleasing ratio is maintained at 1.618.

From what we have learned here, we know we cannot target our fat loss. To sculpt our bodies we must first reduce our overall fat. Then for shaping we can target our shoulders until we reach that magical ratio of 1.618 ratio between shoulders and waist. Then when the boys get out of the shower, they can pull their stomach in, puff out the shoulders and ask, "do I look good". Or some other such narcissistic thing that we all do; at least I hope it's not just me.

GENETICS

Like your height (80%), your weight is 70% determined by your genes as we know from twins and adoption studies.[13] So, that makes our challenge greater as we only have 30% to play with. As you will learn later, the genetic influence is less than this in early life but increases with every decade. I never said this was going to be easy, but the fact that the obesity epidemic is of recent onset means we have very many powerful tools to play with when whispering to our hormones.

SHOES, BOOZE AND MOOBS

Men that drink, particularly heavy beer drinkers all start to look alike. The reason is swelling of the parotid and salivary glands, as well as facial and head fat. Yes, your face and scalp get fatter as you pile on the weight. Your hats have not shrunk. Facial features, like dimples and jaw shape are lost as Jerry and Mike look like Brian, who in turn looks like Dermot.

As you lose weight your shoes will become like boats, as your feet lose fat. New shoes please.

When a crash diet occurs, or you're holed up in bed with flu and not eating for 2 days, you can calculate your liver glycogen storage by your weight loss, assuming you have managed to get 2-3 liters of fluid in per day, which is recommended. Because glycogen requires 3 molecules of water for storage, if you lose 2 kg, by dividing your weight loss by 4, bingo the answer, in this case 0.5 kg, is your total glycogen stored. The moment you eat any carbohydrates it simply returns; your glycogen returns with the water and the 2 kg are back.

As well as obesity, estrogen is also increased in men by stress and liver disease and excessive alcohol consumption. This leads to decreased erectile function, decreased libido and clotting disorders. These effects of estrogen are reduced in both sexes by exercise and in women has been associated with reduced risk of breast cancer. It should also be noted that man boobs are associated with drug use, both prescription and illegal. So, marijuana, methadone, heroin, amphetamine join alcohol as precursors of man boobs, or moobs.

CHAPTER WHISPERINGS

- Fat comes of all over and fat loss cannot be targeted

- Endurance training is not associated with weight loss in non-athletes

- Exercise and weight training are great for health, but not weight loss

- Muscle has three fiber types, slow-twitch, fast-twitch-I and fast-twitch-II

- Resistance training of fiber types causes growth by 0% in ST, 25% in FT-I and 100% in FT-II

- Endurance trained limbs do not build large muscle mass

- Leg cellulite is reduced by endurance running

- The Golden ratio of 1.618 is a perfect aspect seen throughout nature

- Heavy drinking makes us lose our facial features

- Moobs are caused by alcohol and other drugs

- When we lose weight is come off everywhere including our feet and head

CHAPTER 13

THE SUGAR, FAT AND YOGURT WAR

"For every complex problem there is an answer that is clear, simple and wrong"

H.L. Mencken

INTRODUCTION

The Swiss eat cheese like it's going out of fashion. Who else would melt a pound of Gruyere in front of a fire, scrape it off and then use a fondue fork to dip bread into it until it's all gone! And in southwestern France, the Gascons feast on their beloved Garbure, Magret and Confit de Canard; forget living off the fat of the land, this is living off the fat of the table. And these folks have some of the longest life expectancy in Europe.

Over a decade ago, I cycled the tow-path of the canal-du-midi from Toulouse to its end in the beautiful town of Marseillan, a port town on the Etang-du-Thau. A wonderful trip with friends and family. We had parked the car in Toulouse and would five days later would return by train. In 1681, the canal's builder Pierre-Paul Riquet had lined the tow-path with ancient Plane trees giving it a unique and characteristic beauty. The trees provide dappled shade from the baking sun and their roots cause incursions that corrugate the towpath, providing a test for the most cushioned of cycling shorts. Richella, Monique's sister was on that trip, knowing she was terminally ill and died later that year. We miss her.

Instead of driving home from Toulouse, Monique and I headed south into Gascony. Our base was to be Le Bastard Hotel in Lectoure; a small but typical bastide town, with its own cathedral and nestled up on a hill in the Northern Gascony or Gers as it is now known. I need no excuse to visit, but this time it was to find a good Madiran wine. It is dark red and so rich in polyphenols that I fancied I would make my fortune importing this miraculous wine. Many bottles were imported but were also drank at parties at home with friends. In spite of my penchant for keeping very expensive and fine wines bought en-primeur, I was hapless with the cheaper Madirans. I had discovered also, an aerator device that instantly brought these young wines to their fruitiest best, and it made a wonderful sucking noise to boot. I bought as many as the shop had and gave them to my friends at home as presents.

We arrived very tired and went straight to bed. We awoke to the fabulous views and the smells of Gascony. That Sunday morning, we had a lie in, then wondered around the town and found a bar for a drink. It was narrow fronted with a few tables outside, but long, dark and earthy inside. It had a long thin bar on the left and stretched back to a kitchen. It's shape made the staff more frenetic than they would have to be in a more ergonomically shaped saloon. We sat at a table midway down, on the right, backs against the wall, and in that foreign bar sort of way, not quite sure whether to wait or go to the bar. The barman was rushing between the few chairs and tables in the street to the kitchen. The food menu was on a blackboard and in spite of good French neither of us could fathom a single word. A guy came to sit at the table next to us, with a girl pierced, tattooed and filled with melancholy. She was nonetheless attractive in a French, Betty Blue sort of way. He sat down awkwardly, until he removed his hunting knife from his midriff, and thrust it into the table. Wow. This was very earthy indeed. I ordered two beers at the bar pronto, and as usual got short-changed. It was a strange place, but a few beers later, I'd acclimatized to the knife. At regular intervals a girl would emerge from the kitchen, at first with bread, and then other foodstuffs, slapping them onto customer's tables, with little finesse. We knew it was from an animal, as there is no "V" in the Gascon dictionary. Serve Gascons vegetarian food, they just shrug their shoulders in that Gallic, laconic sort of way.

The food was unrecognizable by look, smell or taste. It was like a gnarled mound of cold burger; fist sized and dark brown. Johnny Gascon on my left, used his dagger to slice it for him and Betty Blue. Monique and I nibbled at the edges of this huge mound of cold hard thing. It tasted interesting, but strangely got better the more we ate. For two days we breathed, belched and sweated that stuff. God only knows what it was, but it lingered for sure. You see, that's the Gascons; they live in towns built on hills, go to church and shrug their shoulders a lot. They eat very odd diets, huge in animal fats, and live to a ripe old age.

THE ANTI-FAT-EATERS

The anti-fat-eating brigade suggest that the Swiss get protection from altitude, and Gascons protection from their local wines. But this ignores the fact that four fifths of Swiss live in the lowlands and the argument that one single protective factor protects the Gascons, is just too simple*.

This whole anti-fat thing came from transatlantic scientific hypotheses and studies in the 1960s. Heart disease was a new thing that century and was on the up. Medicine and governments needed to know why. The two counter arguments could not have been clearer; the Brits said it was sugar and the US argued it was fats. In reading this very sentence, examine your own bias. If you have been alive for any of the last 60 years, you will have been indoctrinated like the rest of us. I'm afraid to say, we have been force fed the deplorable nonsense that fat is bad.

*Red Madiran wines have four times the number of heart protecting polyphenols. The local terroir is highly suited to the Tannat grape, producing a deep dark earthy red, best aerated into a decanter and drunk medium young at 17-18 C. A truly delicious accompaniment to any high-fat diet.

THE TRANSATLANTIC FAT VERSUS SUGAR WAR. THE WINNERS WERE CORPORATE FOOD. THE LOSERS WERE US.

In the USA, Ansell Keys was convincing the Americans that a low-fat diet was the right way. In England, John Yudkin was arguing that it was sugar that was the devil, and we should reduce our refined and super-refined carbohydrates.

The greatest controversy in world of nutrition is the work of Ansel Keys. An American, who with his wife, latterly described the Mediterranean diet. He went on to die at the age of 100 in 2004, in the same year as his wife, in his beloved Italy. He leaves two children, one of whom is a physician. The third child was tragically shot during a burglary in the US aged 42.

The source of the Keys controversy was that Keys first proposed that saturated animal fat was correlated with heart disease. In the 1960s, heart disease was a new problem and of increasing concern to governments in the West, and particularly in the US. Keys embarked on the "20 countries study", presenting correlations between the intake of animal saturated fats and "reported" (and that's an important word) blood vessel atheromatous heart disease at death.

Yudkin, had contemporaneously, produced a book named "Pure, White and Deadly" (1972), a book about the evils of sugar. He argued that it was the rise in sugar consumption that was causing the cardiac problems. Many of the problems associated with sugar were later brilliantly detailed in Robert Lustig's book, "Fat Chance; The Hard Truth about Sugar, Obesity and Disease." Dr Lustig is a pediatric endocrinologist, who outlines with clarity and wisdom the influences that sugar and hormones have on our ill-health.[31] Like me, he believes that sugar is as dangerous to us as cigarettes. Strong stuff from a man of letters.

The argument goes like this. Keys argued that the cause of ischemic heart disease was down to consumption of saturated animal fats. There was much peer criticism when he presented it at the WHO, and much criticism over the accuracy of his epidemiological statistics; in particular correlation versus causation. Oddly, he also reduced the study from his original hypothesis of twenty countries to seven. I don't know why Keys reduced the number of countries in his study, and none of us can ever know. What we do know, is there are other sources of bias too. For example, the recorded cause of death is wildly inaccurate, both within and between nations. We know that estimates of fat consumption have many biases; including increased waste in more affluent countries. His own raw data shows a negative correlation between high saturated fat consumption and overall mortality. In other words, saturated fat consumption correlates with lower death rates from all causes. Many others have questioned the conclusions Keys drew from his own data.[119] Others have rightly questioned the whole concept of replacing fats with carbohydrates, in low-fat food.[120] After all, heart disease was new, we were well into the second carbohydrate revolution and awash with sugar and had been eating high fat diets since the start of time.

THE RESULT OF KEYS' WORK

The day that Ansel Keys finally persuaded the politicians running the senate committee on Diet and Nutrition, that food must contain less fat, the world fell into perilous times. And it was really easy to get the corporates and farmers on board because it would be;

- a revolution in the food industry and

- America's farming belt was now producing millions of acres of corn, from which the sugar substitute, High Fructose Corn Syrup is made

The food corporates went to work, removing the fat from everything we eat. Order a new private jet they shouted. The fat cats would have their day. "Let's remove all the fat from all the food" they roared. And so, the food scientists found ways of removing fat from food. When fat is removed from, yogurt, cheese, breakfast cereal, milk, in fact anything and everything, you get low-fat versions of the same. The hideous world of "low-fat" food was born. But the biggest hurdle lay ahead.

LOW FAT YOGURT

When the fat was taken it out, the yogurt tasted bad. So bad that low-fat yogurt resembled wallpaper paste, with the wallpaper paste removed. The corporate jets were cancelled. How could the scientists catch up with their marketing departments? Much head scratching and back to the drawing board.

Eureka. Why not replace the fat in food with sugar? The food boffins tried this one and the taste was great. Arguably better than with the original fat still in it. But when the corporate bean counters did the maths, the yogurt would cost the same as the jet!

A CHANCE MEETING THAT WRECKED THE WORLD

On an internal flight heading home for Thanksgiving, two Americans would meet by sheer coincidence. They introduced themselves and no doubt asked about each other's salaries. Once the unpleasantries were over they got talking about what they did, in that most un-English sort of way. When an Englishman travels, a polite nod of the head before disembarkation is sufficient communication with your neighboring passenger.

Peter was based in the Mid-West and told his stories of how there was a glut in corn. The other told his story of how his company had charged him with the challenge of removing fat from food. The two of them chatted away on the flight. Jim explained that the solution was to add sugar and the taste was great. The problem with low-fat yogurt, was not the taste, but the cost. His new best friend Peter explained that they should use high fructose corn syrup, which was a byproduct of the corn industry. Very sweet, but cheap as chips.

In one chance meeting, on one airplane, the low-fat food industry was born. Ever since the low-fat food industry marketing departments have been telling us that low-fat foods help us lose weight and make us healthier. They don't! They fill us with fructose, make us fatter, unhealthier and kill us prematurely. Most importantly, you now that now.

Whilst owners, scientists and managers entered corporate Nirvana, the rest of us were about to lose control of our hormones for 50 years. We were climbing on board the inflammation bus, that would pass the stops of obesity, metabolic syndrome, diabetes, cardiovascular disease and cancer, on route to an early demise. Take your chance to get off ASAP. Anyone for a low-fat yogurt?

READ THE LABEL

Firstly, I wouldn't eat this stuff, but if you do you should always read the label. The crafty corporates use so many names to disguise the sugar that they add to foods to get you hooked. Buyer beware. The names of sugar include;

Agave nectar, Beet sugar, Blackstrap molasses, Brown sugar, Buttered syrup, Cane juice crystals, Cane sugar, Caramel, Carob syrup, Castor sugar, Coconut sugar, Crystalline fructose, Date sugar, Demerara sugar, D-ribose Galactose, Evaporated cane juice, Florida crystals, Fructose, Fruit juice, Fruit juice concentrate, Golden sugar, Golden syrup, Grape sugar, HFCS (high fructose corn syrup), Honey Icing sugar, Maple syrup Molasses, Muscovado sugar, Panela sugar, Raw sugar, Refiner's syrup, Sorghum syrup, Sucanat, Sucrose (table sugar), Treacle sugar, Turbinado sugar, Yellow sugar, Barley malt, Brown rice syrup, Corn syrup, Corn syrup solids, Dextrin, Dextrose, Diastatic, malt Ethyl, maltol ,Glucose, Glucose solids, Lactose, Malt syrup, Maltodextrin, Maltose, Rice syrup.

Eating natural foods which contain sugars is fine. The soft and hard fiber with protect you from the sugar rush and the insulin spike and the subsequent hypoglycemia associated with the soda drink syndrome we met earlier.

FRUCTOSE

The fructose in high fructose corn syrup (HFCS) is indicated by its suffix number. So HFCS55 is 55% fructose and 45% glucose. HFCS45 is used in foodstuffs like breakfast cereals and HFCS55 is used in soft drinks like the soda drinks we talked about earlier. Glucose when consumed is burned and any excess converted into muscle or liver glycogen. The real problems with fructose are that it causes many health problems. Excess fructose is converted into fats in the liver, damages glucose metabolism, causes insulin resistance and increases the aging process through the Maillard process. It also damages liver mitochondria. It causes non-alcoholic fatty liver disease and increases hunger by leptin resistance. You have been warned, avoid it.

CHAPTER WHISPERINGS

- The Swiss and Gascons enjoy diets rich in fats and live to a ripe old age
- Ansel Keys reduced his 20 countries study to 7 for no known reason
- Ansel Keys argued in favour of diets low in saturated animal fat
- John Yudkin knew it was sugar that was killing us, but was ignored
- Low-fat foods are associated with weight gain, not loss
- Many low-fat foods use HFCS as the preferred sugar
- HFCS causes obesity and all the consequences
- HFCS causes aging of body tissues
- HFCS causes leptin resistance and hunger
- Low-fat foods with added sugar make us hungry
- Low-fat foods with added sugar cause our body's insulin hormone to lay down fat and lock fat into our body stores
- High fat foods do not do this, but allow us to burn fat

CHAPTER 14

DIET MYTHOLOGY

"Insanity is doing the same thing over and over and expecting a different result."

Albert Einstein.

INTRODUCTION

As science has proven, both the weight loss and benefits of diets are nullified at one year.[121] Diets do not work, and Einstein was correct about insanity; the business model for most diet companies is a model of quick win, long-term failure and transfer your money to their bank account; and repeat. Diets do not work. If you like the diet club because it gives you social connectivity and you've made friends, I totally get that; there is a strong correlation between community and longevity. But let's not fool anyone, it is not the road to a permanent and sustainable weight loss and good health. Keep going to the diet club if you so wish, but let's get down to the serious business of weight loss and better mental and physical health; and we'll debunk some mythology on the way.

THE 1ST MYTH: DIETS WILL HELP YOU TO LOSE WEIGHT

Diets do not work. This year in the British Medical Journal, Ling Ge published a peer reviewed paper reviewing 121 trials of 21,942 patients.[80] This metanalysis compared all popular macronutrient diets, such as low-fat, low-carbs and calorie restricting with a normal diet. At 6 months, all diets showed modest weight reduction and reduced blood pressure. At 12 months, weight reduction and improvements in cardiovascular risk, had diminished. The exception was reduced LDL cholesterol still evident at 12 months in the Mediterranean diet.

149

THE 2ND MYTH: WE BURN OFF OUR FAT

The truth is, you breathe out the metabolized fat as carbon dioxide. So, when you lose weight you breathe it out, and pee some out as well. We tend to think when we burn something it disappears, but this is incorrect. Fat has a mass and there is a law in physics called "the conservation of mass". Which means that when we burn things they don't disappear. The total mass of the products after "burning" are the same as the total mass of the reactants at the beginning. So, burning doesn't make things disappear, it merely rearranges them into other forms.

The sun's energy is transferred to carbon dioxide and water to create the nutrients in plants or indirectly the animals we eat. After eating our fats, carbs and proteins, we store them or use them for metabolism. When we metabolize fat, we recover the sun's energy from the foods we previously ate. The food is used to make the ATP energy tokens, that power our body. When we metabolize fat, water and carbon dioxide are produced. Water is lost in urine, feces, tears and sweat. Carbon dioxide is breathed out (figure 14.1). So ultimately, we use energy to propel ourselves and that energy came from the sun.

When 10 Kg of fat is lost it produces some 8.40 Kg of carbon dioxide and 1.60 Kg of water. This was the conclusion from a paper by Meerman and Brown.[122] Their appreciation of physics and stoichiometry stretched my memory to beyond its Madiran pickled limits of high school Maths, Physics and Chemistry. And this is interesting although the authors acknowledge there are some limitations in applying physics to the human body. That is because the human body is not a closed system, and fat produces ketone bodies and glucose that are also available for metabolism. The other missing factor is hormones, which is why the calorie counting fails.

Burning fat is a good phrase that is used widely, and we use it too; but it is an analogy rather than actually happens.

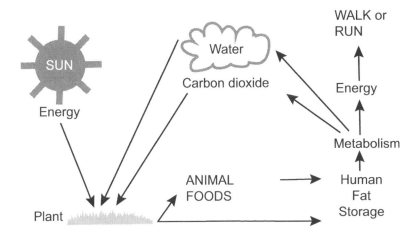

Figure 14.1. Carbon dioxide and water use the sun's energy to produce plants. This then eaten, stored and the metabolism of stored fat, releases energy, water and carbon dioxide. Ultimately, we use the suns energy to power us.

THE 3ᴿᴰ MYTH: CALORIE COUNTING

The whole basis of the calorie counting argument is flawed. We are told that if we reduce our calories, we will lose weight. We are told over and over again that calories in = calories out. And, if our calories going in are less than those going out, you will lose weight. You've heard them all. And guess what? None of them work in real life!

The reason that reducing calories doesn't work is two things. Firstly, your hormones have a primary reason to be; their raison d'etre. To protect your body from yourself, they will make you hungry, cold and miserable. They will make you tired and sleepy and slow down your heart and make you grumpy. Secondly, under these hormonal effects, you will need a will of iron to face that lettuce leaf on your plate. It will be a matter of time until you're off to the burger bar.

This is called hormonal homeostasis. Which literally means your hormones "keeping you the same". They've done that for every generation above you. And, they're not about to change. Which brings me to our next myth.

THE 4ᵀᴴ MYTH: THE 1ST LAW OF THERMODYNAMICS CAN BE APPLIED TO THE BODY

This law states that "in a closed system, energy cannot either be created nor destroyed in a closed system, but merely changed to another form". It is often quoted in reference to calorie counting diets, but guess what, the human body is not a "closed system".

The human body is different from simple thermodynamics (Energy in = Energy out). And, the reason is hormones. The body is as stubborn as it is clever. It makes its mind up and says yep, this guy should be 213 pounds (c. 97 kg). In our desire to be thinner, we look down on our body, hormones and brain, like we are somehow the ones in control. We all do it. We think, this is simple; as long as energy in is less than energy out, we will lose weight. Sure, physics is physics, but it just won't help you to lose weight.

We lose weight initially, then just when we think we're winning, boom we hit a plateau. The weight just stops shedding. Our hormones turn down our metabolism. Slow the heart, makes us tired and sleep more. They will make us feel hungry and grumpy. They will do everything in their power to get us back to the pizza house. Time is the great leveler, and just like the odds on the roulette table, the longer you play, the more likely the house will win. Only your body is the house and your hormones the quietly spoken croupier.

In his brilliant book on fasting, Fung makes a beautiful analogy of short-termism in measuring the success or failure of diets.[123] Like putting water on an iron pipe and looking for rust; you put it on for a day, no rust. Two, three days, three weeks, still nothing. Only after 12 months can the pipe be seen to have been badly corroded by the water". As Fung says, short term weight loss studies just don't cut it with him, and nor do they with me. Study after study, show that weight will return to normal if the hormones are not addressed. Which brings me to our next myth, about how much influence we really have over our weight.

THE 5TH MYTH: WEIGHT IS A MATTER OF CHOICE

In the study of nature versus nurture, there are two classic opportunities.

1. Study identical and non-identical twins, as they are 100% and 50% genetically similar respectively. The similarity of non-identical twins is the same as normal siblings, and they may of course, as normal siblings may, be different sexes.

2. Study identical twins split at birth who were adopted into different families.

Professor Robert Plomin has devoted his life to the study of twins. His latest book "Blueprint" is brilliant and on our suggested reading list.[13] In looking at how our genes influence behavior and our bodies, some things seem logical and intuitive. What is truly amazing is how wrong we can all be, when the science defies what we truly believe. Professor Plomin asked 5000 people some questions about a whole range of physical and mental attributes. If you want to play this game, then it is important you do not skip this bit and peep at the data below. I was wildly wrong and so was Monique!

Firstly, let me explain genetic heredity. If you score eye color with 95% heredity, you'd be right. This means that 95% of the differences between peoples' eye color can be attributed to differences in their DNA. This also means that 5% of the differences are due to environmental factors. So, if I were to ask you for the percentage for genes versus environment in the following, you can write these down. For a bit of fun ask your family too.

1. Breast cancer

2. Height

3. Weight

4. School achievement

5. Autism

6. Spatial ability

The answers are at the end of the paragraph. How did you do?

The three facts that stood out to us were;

- One is that a gene is more prevalent in some people with obesity, that helps to store fat. This was of considerable use to our ancestors where food was scarce, making the gene more likely to survive through to modern humans. It is now considerably less useful to those living where cheap food is plentiful

- The second is that weight is 70% hereditary. So, the differences in people's weight is 70% genetic and 30% environmental

- This genetic heritability increases over time. So, even if you don't resemble your family's weight at 4 years old (40% hereditary), when you're in your middle years (60%) and when you're about to take your pension it will be nearer 80%. Truly fascinating.

The answers to the above were 1. 10% 2. 80% 3. 70% 4. 60% 5. 70% 6. 70%.

Surprised? I was and if you are now thinking twice about school fees or whether civilian pilots are assessed for spatial orientation, I'm with you. And, you know where to read more.[13]

So, whatever your genes are doing, we still have 30% to play with. It also important to remember that we have other enemies lurking in our fight against the flab and our genes;

- Hormones and hormonal homeostasis

- Corporate fast food scientists searching for that "bliss point" on your taste buds

- Corporate marketing; you need breakfast, three meals a day, this takeaway, that takeaway, this snack etc.

- Fast food delivery companies, tempting you every time you sit down

- Chefs adding sweetness to almost every food, getting you sugar addicted and turning on your fat fuel inhibition

So, if you've found your clothes shrinking, or your scales are incorrect, we can work together on that 30%. It is far from hopeless once you learn to whisper your hormones back into shape, getting you back in control.

THE 6TH MYTH: YOU CAN WEIGHT TRAIN YOUR WAY OUT OF THE KITCHEN

By now you'll know that both Monique and I do a mix of resistance training, running, cycling and swimming. Hopefully, it offsets some of our fun foods and drink. Fewer bullets flying at us, rather than all or none. Building muscle is a healthy thing to do. It not only makes us feel a lot better but will help to combat the natural aging muscle wastage. So, do not mistake the message here. Muscle is great, it's just the outrageous gym adverts that make us smile. If you read the gym adverts, you'll come across these three gems; so spectacular, they qualify for the whisperer "Equine Effluent Awards".

- The best of all are the outrageous claims is "what muscle building can do to boost your metabolism". In our body's furnace our body's energy burn is; liver 25%, brain 20%, muscles 15%; kidneys 10%, heart 10% and the other 20% is spread amongst skin, gut, lungs and fat. Muscle is about 3 times more metabolically active that fat. Our lean tissue is around 80%, with 20% being fat. In a 200-pound man (90kg or 14 stone), a ten per cent gain in muscle from weight training would required a significant training commitment. This would result in a 16 pounds (c. 7 kg) increase in muscle mass. If his BMR were 2000 calories per day, his muscle burn per day would be 300 calories. This new muscle will not revolutionize his metabolism. Instead, it will burn a measly 30 calories or 1/10th of a snicker bar.

- "After-burn from HIIT will be your savior and burn thousands of calories". Sorry folks, but that is so minor it really accounts for very little, at about 4% of your BMR. Minute for minute HIIT is slightly better than cardio, but taking into account the longer cardio, overall effects are similar and singularly unimpressive compared to the hype.

- There is little after-burn after resistance training. After a 40-minute session there may be 4% or 80 calories of increase over 24 hours. Wow, a quarter of that snicker bar.[124]

These are piffling amounts; our diet is by far the most powerful tool in reducing calorific balance. Please do the cardio, the HIIT and the weights, because you like it, and they're good for you. At least you won't be one of the fools believing and even worse repeating this hype.

THE 7TH MYTH: YOU CAN OUTRUN YOUR KITCHEN

Let me start by saying there are some exceptional athletes that can. They are able to exercise for hour after hour and include cross-country skiers, endurance cyclists and ultra-runners.

The more you exercise, the more your hormones slow down your resting BMR. So, one week you go to the gym every day and do your "cardio" and run for 1 hour on the treadmill. You're doing it well and mixing up the slow and long and HIIT 80/20, and I've been there too. Two hours slogging my 213 pounds (c. 97 kg) over a rotating rubber band. And in the background my hormones are waiting their moment. When we sit down in the afternoon, they slow down my resting metabolism, make me tired, fall to sleep and feel hungry and grumpy. They know that I cannot do anymore in the gym than two hours cardio, which burns 1200 Kcal. I've got 2 hours to increase my BMR and beat them, and the hormones have the other 22 hours to slow down by BMR and make sure I lose. We know that fat becomes more metabolically active with exercise, but just does not get burned off.[125] You have to be a very special athlete to outrun your hormones and be pretty lean already. And the higher proportion of body fat the worse this phenomenon.

THE 8TH MYTH: YOU CAN OUTRUN YOUR HORMONES

Your see the hormones do very crafty things to scupper those calorie counting diets. By definition, you came from ancestors that could survive in harsh periods of food deprivation and were better at escaping the saber-toothed tigers than the bloke in the next cave. And on an empty belly. They could hunt and fought successfully against their enemies, all on an empty belly. If they couldn't, they wouldn't have survived, and you wouldn't be here. So, you descend from survivors, whose hormones knew how to keep them alive, in times of food scarcity. When they had no food, the hormones knew their body's metabolism needed to be shut down, to preserve energy. You are now that person living in a world replete with food.

What happens is the process of self-preservation, hard-wired into you for hundreds of generations above you. It's called homeostasis and its controlled by hormones and its rock-hard and stubborn as hell. In those days it was survival of the fittest; now it's survival of the smartest.

CHAPTER WHISPERINGS

- Diets do not work if you watch them for long enough
- The Mediterranean diet is associated with lowering bad LDL cholesterol
- When we lose 10 kg of fat it is metabolized into 8.4 kg of carbon dioxide and 1.6 kg of water, resulting in 10 kg of weight loss
- Calorie counting does not work to lose weight because of hormones and metabolism
- Weight is 70% inherited and varies in time; lower as children and slightly higher as we get older
- Our 30% environmental factors for weight, vary in time and place
- Only supreme endurance athletes can outrun their kitchens
- Building 10% more muscle is worth about 1/10th of a snicker bar per day
- Resistance training sessions produce 24 hours of piffling afterburn worth ¼ snicker bar
- There is the same 24 hour after-burn following HIIT and cardio and not very much in either
- Your hormones have been keeping you safe for millennia. Work with them for total control of your weight, hitting targets and staying there

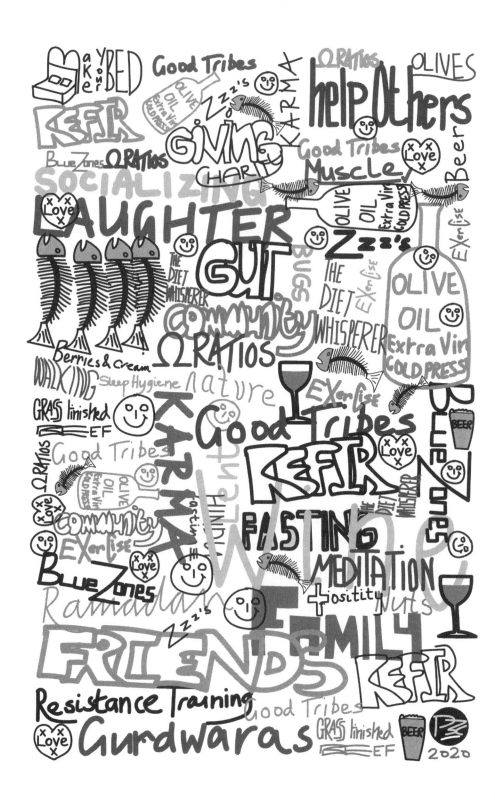

PART TWO

THE ROAD TO PERMANENT WEIGHT LOSS

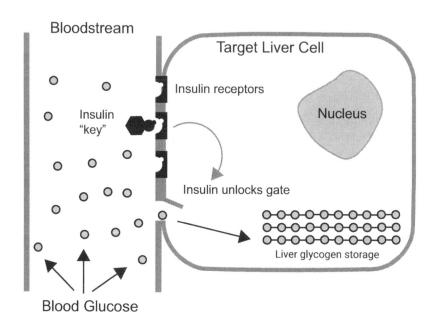

Figure 15.1. Raised blood glucose, releases insulin, which binds to its receptors in the cell wall. This causes the gate to open in the cell wall, letting glucose into cells and stimulates glycogen production in liver and muscle cells.

CHAPTER 15

HORMONES MADE SIMPLE

"Eureka, I have found it."

Archimedes

INTRODUCTION

During this chapter, you will have a Eureka moment. I'd like to start with some fantastic news. Although there are over 50 hormones, you only need to know a lot about one, and a little about another four.

In his Croonian lecture, at The Royal College of Physicians in 1905 Ernest Starling, Professor of physiology at University College London, presented the word "hormone". Hormone is from the Greek "to set in motion", and is quite simply a chemical messenger, produced by one type of cell, enters the bloodstream, where it travels to exert an effect on another distant cell. They recognize their target cells by the receptors, usually found within the cell wall of the target cell (figure 15.1).

WHAT ARE HORMONES?

Hormones are tiny chemical messengers in the blood stream. Imagine a letter your postman delivers. The letter is written (produced), posted and then travels by road and is delivered to the target cell, your house. When it reaches your door, it exerts a target effect on the cell, in this case your house, or the people within it. If it's your bank manager informing you that your life savings are missing, the target effect will be chaos in the house. A reasonable question would be why not use the telephone, the equivalent of our nervous system? And the answer is that 100,000 other cells (houses) had their savings stolen at the same time, and he wanted to communicate with them all at the same time. In other words, hormones enable thousands of target cells to be affected simultaneously. In the body our hormones are pretty quick, hitting their target cells within 10 seconds. A bit faster than snail mail.

If it's a letter from your new lover, it will have a positive effect on the target cell, and there will be much joy and perhaps even music and dancing. The road the letters travel on, is like the bloodstream for our hormones. When you received the love letter, you may have felt a flutter in your stomach. That is partly your vagus nerve that connects your brain to your gut and partly hormones released by the brain. So, it's the nervous system and the hormonal system, working in harmony to keep us alive and give us our pleasures. A chemical called dopamine increases in your brain. And your pituitary gland in the skull, releases oxytocin into the blood, which amongst other things is our human-to-human bonding hormone. If you love your partner just as much as ever but wonder why you don't get that fluttery feeling anymore, don't worry. It's natural after a few years that this hormonal release slows, even when the love remains.

Let's take our analogy a step further. A mailbox is too universal, with all letters passing through it. And occasionally, I get the odd letter in my mailbox for George next door and vice versa. This is fine because George and I will pop the letter to its rightful recipient at the earliest. But we need a system whereby George cannot accidentally see that I've been caught speeding again. So rather than letters and a mailbox, the postman uses keys, which fit one of some 52 key holes in each front door. Each key is specific and when turned, creates the target effect in the house automatically. So, the blue key automatically says the occupant's money has been stolen, and the same chaos ensues. The red key sends the same messages from the lover, and there is music and dancing. Every cell has a unique set of key holes for many different keys. Far away an endocrine gland will be posting its unique key into the blood, where they will search for the cells with the right keyhole, so they may exert their target effect. If that key goes to a house without the keyhole for it, the key just won't work.

THE ENDOCRINE SYSTEM

Our endocrine system produces our 52 unique hormones, or keys; made in different glands all over the body. They travel in the blood to exert their unique effect on the target cell. Numerous target cells clumped together are called target tissue, like muscle, and numerous tissues clumped together are called a target organ like the brain, liver or kidney. It is these hormones that fly around our body at all times controlling our metabolism. All day, all night, doing their stuff, from controlling our blood sugar to controlling our sleep.

In the correct terminology, endocrine glands release hormones into the blood, where they travel to exert a unique effect on target cells, tissues or organs. Hormones regulate many of our body's functions. They regulate our development prior to birth and are responsible for ensuring we have two thumbs and eight fingers. After birth, they control our growth, start puberty, and take us through it. They control our immune system and decide who gets facial hair and who doesn't, as well as all the other sexual characteristics. The adrenal glands pump out adrenaline and cortisol when we are in danger, so we can fight or flight. Our kidney creates erythropoietin, that stimulates new red blood cell production, and is on the doping list of all sports for obvious reasons. And insulin, king of hormones to any diet-whisperer, is produced in the pancreas and released into the blood after we eat. It facilitates the transfer of glucose, fats and proteins from the blood into our tissues. Of particular interest to us, is its action on carbohydrates and fats. Insulin is primarily known for its association with glucose and diabetes. But is has another vitally important function, which is fat storage. In my medical schooldays, it was also known as the fat storage hormone.

Hormones control metabolism, speeding it up when we get cold, burning fat as fuel for our body's internal heater. Conversely, hormones slow down our metabolism when we diet and after exercise, to conserve our macronutrient stores. Hormones are our autopilot; they will always work to keep us in balance. Their primary function is keeping us safe and alive. Start the latest trendy diet and our hormones will react. Eat less, and they will slow our metabolism and our heart. They will make us feel tired, lethargic and miserable. So, when you reduce your calories, your hormones

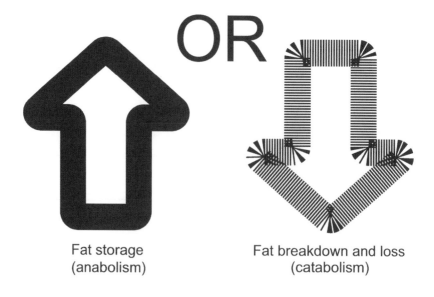

Fat storage
(anabolism)

Fat breakdown and loss
(catabolism)

Figure 15.2.   Hormone driven anabolism (building and storing macronutrients), vs catabolism (breaking down or burning macronutrient stores). They are either one "or" the other and cannot co-exist. You're either storing fat or losing fat. Never both at the same time. And, if insulin is circulating, you are anabolic.

won't approve, because they think food is scarce, and they want you to stay alive. Hormones love things not changing; hormones love things staying the same. It's called hormonal homeostasis. It has meant your ancestors survived for 200,000 years and passed their successful hormones on to you; the ones with poor hormones aren't here. They didn't survive that cold spell in the cave, when there was no food. They couldn't run or fight on an empty stomach. Hormones are well versed, and in the modern world still hold firm their ancient ways, as they know what works well. Because of this, hormones are tricky fellows to beat. So, don't ignore them or shout at them, because they will win. You will learn to control them by whispering gently to get them on your side. They don't like sudden change and by sudden, I mean thousands of years. They prefer to do what they have done for hundreds of generations. And that's how you keep them onside. Do what they know and what they like.

MUTUALLY EXCLUSIVE

Of our 52 hormones keeping us alive, certain hormones control our body's macronutrient metabolism. The macronutrient we're really interested in is fat, because that's what we all want to lose as we shed weight. Think of it this way; on a cold day you put on your clothes to go out. When you come in, you take your clothes off. Both acts of dressing and undressing are mutually exclusive. In other words, you are either putting clothes on or taking clothes off; never both at the same time.

With respect to body fat, certain hormones are anabolic; that is, they cause fat to be stored and increase our body fat. Other hormones are catabolic; that is, they cause fat to be removed from the body, and we reduce our body fat. And these hormones are mutually exclusive; in other words, at any given time, our bodies are either gaining fat, or losing fat (figure 15.2).

If you have circulating insulin, the major anabolic fat storing hormone, you cannot break down fat for fuel. Not now, not tonight, not ever! This point is fundamental to understanding your fat metabolism. If insulin is present in the blood you are laying down fat. If you want to remove fat, insulin must not be present. Only when insulin is absent can the catabolic hormone glucagon, start melting away your body fat.

For a lot of people, this is when the penny drops! When there is raised blood insulin, fat cannot be used for fuel. After eating, insulin will be raised for two to three hours in healthy individuals and up to six hours in overweight individuals with metabolic syndrome or diabetes (figure 15.3).

All foods increase insulin and the following graph shows how different macronutrients affect blood insulin levels (figure 15.4). And here's the rub; that chocolate digestive with your elevenses, renders your body anabolic for two hours, until lunch. And then the snack at teatime, before supper, the same. Before you know it, your insulin is raised 24 hours a day. Then you wonder why you're not losing any fat! It's not the number of calories, it's the type of food and the frequency of food. Eureka?

Let's cut to the quick. Frequent meals or snacks, however small, will put your insulin up for most of the day. The only normalized insulin levels will

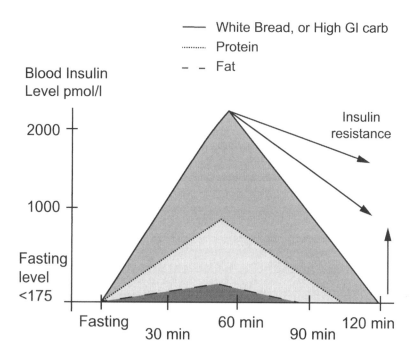

Figure 15.3. Blood insulin after carbohydrate, protein and fat. When insulin resistance, pre-diabetes or diabetes is added; the base of the insulin release widens (see arrows). It shows the differences in the amount of insulin required for different macronutrients. And how much more insulin is secreted when insulin resistance is present.

be overnight. And even then, if you have a bedtime snack, you'll be hours into your sleep before your blood insulin levels fall back to zero. And, dare I mention getting up at night for a snack or soda drink. I'm afraid all of this just puts you right into the epicenter of your own hormonal storm. Not only will you be unable to shift fat, but insulin resistance, metabolic syndrome and diabetes, are lurking just around the corner. Maybe a decade, maybe a year or maybe tomorrow.

Fat causes the lowest insulin release, followed by protein and the highest is unsurprisingly the carbohydrates. And what's worse, the more refined the carbs, the higher the levels. Now you can see the danger in that last thing at night biscuit with your hot chocolate. It's a hormonal car crash. On my 50th

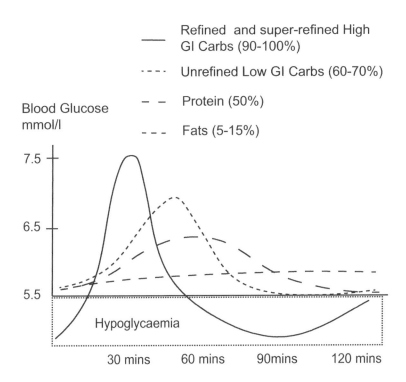

Figure 15.4. Different foods and tendancy for low blood glucose (hypoglycaemia) which then stimulates symptoms of hunger and re-eating. The % figure is the amount converted to glucose. Note: in healthy individuals, hypogycaemia (low blood sugar) only occurs with high GI (refined and super-refined carbs).

birthday, I realized I had to make a choice; booze, puddings or biscuits? The puddings and biscuits lost.

And so, to the corollary; what if we were to eat just one fat filled meal a day? Say, 65% fat, 35% protein and 5% carbohydrates. "That much fat", I hear you say. Well, here lies the truth. Your insulin will hardly rise and will come back to normal after a few hours. The paradox is clear for all to see. If you want to lose weight you have to reduce your insulin. To burn fat, you must have periods when insulin is not in your blood stream. Eat less frequently and you'll burn more fat. Eating fat, causes the burning of fat. And with absolute certainty, cut out all forms of snacking, but particularly with refined and super-refined carbohydrate foods and drinks.

SODA DRINK SYNDROME

Too often we see obese teenagers, walking along, swinging at their side, a 2-liter (c. 4-pints) plastic bottle of soda drink. They keep their soda drink close, to continuously refuel the fire of their sugar addiction; what we call soda drink syndrome (SDS). The teens don't know why they are trapped in this cycle of ever-increasing obesity. They don't need to eat any food to be trapped. They are not only trapped by increasing weight and fat but are laying down new fat cells; something unique to children and adolescents.

Let me terrify you with some figures. We have an orange flavored soda drink in the UK that comes in 2-liter bottles. They cost £1.85 ($ 2.29) and anyone can buy them; and sugar addicted teens frequently do. Each bottle has the equivalent of 71 sugar cubes. Let me tell you how you can work this out simply with some very easy maths.

Soda drinks come with 10 grams of sugar in 100 ml. A sugar cube is 2.8 g, and we know that 1 gram of sugar is 4 calories. So, 2 liters is 2000 ml which is 200 grams of sugar. Multiplying by 4 gives us 800 calories in one bottle. If we divide the 200 by the weight of the sugar cube, we get 71.43 sugar cubes in each bottle.

A teenage girl at 16 has an energy requirement, or BMR, of 1800 calories for the whole day. The worry from these drinks is SDS; a circular pathway which is, have a drink -- spike your blood sugar -- insulin released to chase the rise in blood sugar -- blood sugar rapidly falls -- insulin is still circulating, and the blood sugar falls below the normal level -- and we get symptoms of low blood sugar, a "hypo" or hypoglycemia symptoms; pallor, shakes, irritability, tiredness and lack of concentration - we take another drink. And repeat (figure 15.5).

Even worse the HFCS in this soda drink bottle stimulates another hormone ghrelin, which is our hunger hormone. The HFCS also inhibits our satiety hormone leptin. This results in further hunger for more soda drink. This is SDS and is the cycle of doom. It is refined carbohydrate addiction; it terrifies me that so many teenagers have this. It will, undiagnosed and untreated, lead to a reduced healthspan and lifespan. In other words, they'll

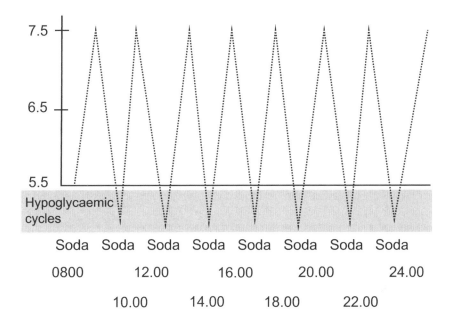

Figure 15.5. Soda Drink Syndrome (SDS). Recurrent spikes in blood sugar followed by recurrent hypos, stimulating the next feed cycle. Super-refined carbs in a bottle.

constantly feel terrible, get horrible inflammatory diseases and die early. More dangerous than cigarettes, and anyone can buy them.

FRUIT JUICE

And now for an even bigger surprise. Fruit juices freshly made, or out of a carton, contain just about the same amount of sugar as soda drinks. The only benefit over the soda drinks is that they contain a few vitamins to boot. Wow, great. Yep, they're just another nonsense that we've been sold as a healthy adjunct to our breakfast. The reason my mother did this for us, was because she didn't know. It wasn't a lack of love; it was a lack of knowledge. This is the very essence of the whisperer family; not dying of ignorance.

When you had your last orange juice, did you feel sleepy an hour or two later? I'd put good money that you did! And the solution? Elevenses, pastry and coffee. Soda Drink Syndrome can be applied to any and every refined and super-refined carbohydrate addiction that we have. Remember, we have 50 times the refined and super-refined carbohydrates in our diet than just 100 years ago. And insulin is there to help us store our un-refined carbohydrates, fats and proteins. It expects to have to hang around for ages as the cabbage and carrots are slowly digested and absorbed. It doesn't expect that blood glucose rush from orange juice or cake. They weren't available to our body's designer. So, it's no surprise that we get those horrible hypoglycemic symptoms after eating this highly refined junk. Hunger is caused by eating carbohydrates. The more refined, the greater the hunger in 1-2 hours' time.

CHAPTER WHISPERINGS

- Hormones are tiny chemical messengers, like keys in the bloodstream
- Hormones attach to target cells, tissues or organs to produce a target action
- Hormones control our metabolism
- Hormonal homeostasis keeps you alive
- Insulin is the hormone of fat storage
- All macronutrients can be stored as fat
- When insulin is present in our blood, we cannot burn fat from our fat stores
- Refined and super-refined carbs lead to higher levels of insulin
- Soda drinks cause hormonal havoc, metabolic syndrome, illness and premature death
- Snacking is bad, snacking with refined carbs is worse and super-refined carbs worse still
- Meal frequency is a massive problem and feeds back on itself
- Junk food, refined and super-refined carbs make us hungry

- Fiber reduces carbohydrate bioavailability and is protective against insulin spikes

- We lose fat only by reducing the amount and circulating time of insulin

- Soda drinks are available to anyone, at any age, but arguably more dangerous than cigarettes

CHAPTER 16

HORMONES AND METABOLISM

"Why are all elderly people so thin? The fat ones didn't make it!"

PBC, diet-whisperer HQ

INTRODUCTION

Our hormones have been regulating our metabolism for the 200,000 years since Homo sapiens evolved. We saw earlier in the food chapter, how we went through the first carbohydrate revolution 12,000 years ago when we started milling flour and introduced refined carbohydrates to the human diet. In the last 100 years, we have entered the second carbohydrate revolution, by increasing our refined carbohydrates and adding in super-refined carbohydrates, such as snacks, pastries, cakes and soda drinks. This has burdened our bodies with a tsunami of sugar, up by 50 times what it was just 100 years ago.

To put this in perspective, let us rebase the timescale of Homo sapiens history from 200,000 years, to 100 years. This means we lived on our familiar diet of unrefined plant vegetables, fruits, fiber and berries to complement our meats for 95 years. So, we lived mainly on fiber, fat and protein for 95 years. Only 5 years ago did we introduce refined carbs. Terrifyingly, that means we've had our super-refined carbs for 18 days. We can easily see that the carbohydrate load is too much for our poor body and hormones to cope with. When I visit my local stores, I genuinely see no difference between the sugary drinks and snacks and the tobacco shelves. The obvious paradox being that children cannot buy the cigarettes.

OUR HORMONES

In the last chapter, we saw that hormones behave like free traveling keys in the bloodstream, looking for the cells that hold a lock for each particular key. And when it finds its lock, the key turns, and the target cell it then instructed to perform a chemical task, dependent on the particular type of key. There is more than one type of receptor on each target cell wall. Depending on the target cell type, there will be receptors for other types of key as well. So, on liver cells for example, we have insulin receptors that open a gate to allow blood glucose into the cell, which is then stored as glycogen. The insulin hormone also stimulates glycogenesis, the restringing of simple glucose molecules into glycogen.

On the same cell wall, we have different receptors for the hormone glucagon; and this does the opposite; stimulating the breakdown of the glycogen chains, or glycogenolysis. Once broken into single glucose units, these are released through gates in the cell wall, and into the blood. The entrance gates from the blood to the cells are opened by insulin, and the release gates from the cell back into the blood are opened by glucagon. And these are mutually exclusive; they cannot happen at the same time.

Our endocrine system detects when blood levels of glucose have increased and releases insulin, and when they fall releases glucagon. This is our hormonal homeostasis, responsible for the management of our blood glucose. And it's important, because if the blood sugar falls to zero, we're dead.

We have seen there are in excess of fifty human hormones circulating in our bodies. It is a veritable soup of biological activity, without which we would be unable to work, rest, eat, breathe or pass on our genes. Working in perfect harmony with our central nervous system, our endocrine system keeps us alive and well.

This soup of hormones controls us in every aspect of our lives, without us ever even being aware of their presence. We can sometime feel the effects of our hormones, like adrenaline, making our hearts pound and pupils dilate, when faced with danger. And, the corollary is also true, that deficiencies can be debilitating or fatal. Patients with a deficiency in adrenal hormones can die very quickly untreated. Growth hormone deficiency leads to "stunted" growth. And before the discovery of the hormone insulin, type 1 diabetes, where insulin is absent, was a lethal condition; an early description of "the body's tissues passing out in the urine". Thirsty patients, frequently passing urine and wasting away until an early death. It can be said that we have had tremendous success in treating hormonal deficiencies over the years, from growth hormone deficiency, through type 1 diabetes with insulin treatment and hormone replacement in post-menopausal women.

But buyer beware, there is no hormone treatment that I can think of that does not have a few or many unwanted side effects. Whilst we know a great deal about what each hormone does, we are far from knowing everything they do. And there are all those new hormone-like peptides around the gut microbiome. Hence, the veritable soup; my way of describing the millions of complex interactions our hormones have with each other and our different body cells, tissues and organs. Not to mention our mental state and emotions. When incretin hormones were first discovered, GIP and GLP-1, a new hope was born for diabetes therapy. The problems encountered were not that they didn't work, but the many other effects these hormones had on the body. A complex soup indeed.

There are four groups of hormones based on their chemical backbones and are classified as amino acids, eicosanoids, peptides and steroids. Chemically they are built from fats or proteins and vary in size and shape, allowing their unique "key" like identification at target cell receptor sites. And surprisingly, from release to target action is only ten seconds; somewhat faster than snail mail.

INSULIN AND GLUCAGON

Insulin was discovered by Banting, Best and Macleod, at the University of Toronto in 1921. Banting and Macleod went on to win the Nobel Prize for Physiology and Medicine in 1923. Insulin is produced in the beta islet of Langerhans's cells in our pancreas and on reaching its target receptors in the cell wall of fat, liver and muscle cells, causes glucose to enter and be stored as glycogen or fat. High blood glucose is the trigger for its release, allowing blood glucose levels to fall, which is its desired effect. When insulin is circulating, fat can only be stored. As long as insulin is present in the blood, fat cannot be broken down.

The role of insulin is to direct macronutrients to where they are needed in the body. When the insulin key is inserted into the receptor cell, carbohydrates, fats and proteins may enter the cell. When we consume super-refined carbohydrates, they do not require any digestion and rush rapidly into the bloodstream. Insulin is released and rapidly moves sugar into target tissues. If you're exercising this may go into muscle for energy production; if you're at your desk, it will be converted into fat stores. The sugar spike caused by the super-refined carbohydrates is soon gone, but the insulin takes longer to disappear. It is used to much slower absorbed foods, like carrots or cabbage. Therefore, as there is insulin but no excess glucose, the insulin causes the blood sugar to fall to below normal, and ghrelin is released causing us to feel rapidly hungry again. This creates that tired, shaky, hypoglycemic sensation 90 minutes after eating refined and super-refined carbohydrates. This keeps us eating and effectively keeps a constant blood insulin and constant fat storage.

Glucagon is a close neighbor of insulin in the alpha islet cells in the pancreas. Its functions are very much as the opposite of insulin. Glucagon is released when blood sugar is low, to protect us from the inevitable damage that would cause. Glucagon causes glucose to be released into the blood to raise our blood glucose levels to a safe level. It does this by glycogenolysis, or the cleaving of stored cell glycogen into glucose and opens the gates to let it out. When glycogen stores run out, glucagon switches on cellular glucose production from fats and proteins; gluconeogenesis. When glucagon is around, fats can be broken down.

The actions of insulin and glucagon are mutually exclusive. In the next chapter we will detail the specific carbohydrate controls that make us ill, but also can make us so much healthier.

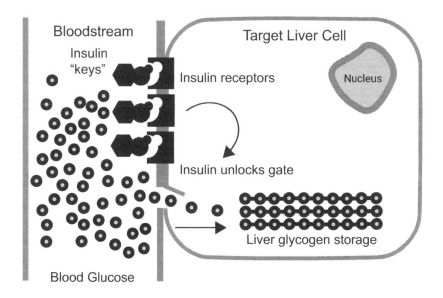

Figure 16.1. Insulin resistance. Sustained high blood glucose, eventually requires more insulin to open cell gates, allowing glucose to move from the blood into liver and muscle cells. Blood glucose and blood insulin are levels are both raised.

INSULIN RESISTANCE

With obesity, firstly comes insulin resistance, then metabolic syndrome, then diabetes, then chronic ill-heath, then an early death. Brutal but true.

Insulin resistance is a key point to understand; it occurs when the hormonal effect of insulin on target cells is diminished. It is caused when insulin is too high for too long. Rather than a cell needing one insulin key to store the glucose as glycogen, it needs two, then three and so on. If there is too much blood glucose emanating from our diet, over time, we will need more and more insulin to move it into the cells. This causes insulin to become less effective. Then, more and more insulin is required, and the pancreas eventually becomes exhausted beyond trying to keep up with an ever-increasing demand. Demand outstrips supply. This situation prevents glucose from being stored in the target cells. Glucose then backs up in the blood, causing raised blood glucose (figure 16.1 and 16.2).

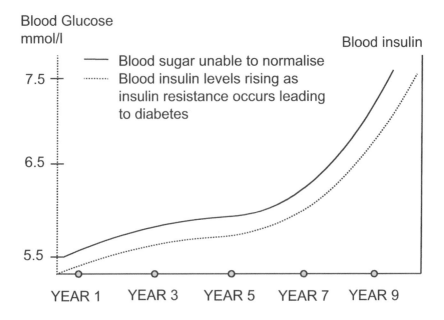

Figure 16.2. Insulin resistance over time, causing raised blood insulin and raised blood glucose.

It comes about with worrying simplicity and symptomless stealth. Insulin resistance is now evident in 100 million Americans! That is 30% of the US population. Genetics and race play a part in the cause of insulin resistance, but again, our interaction with our food and the environment are the big take home messages. Insulin resistance is associated with;

• Race; all races, but with increased risk for Black, south Asian or Hispanic

• Genetics; all races with family history of metabolic syndrome or type 2 diabetes

• In 80% of obese people with time

• Insulin resistance can occur in people with little subcutaneous body fat but increased visceral fat. This is commonly seen in south Asians. Metabolically Obese Normal Weight (MONW) describes this sub-group

• Insulin resistance results from refined and super-refined carbohydrates in the diet

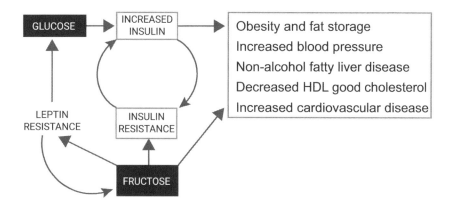

Figure 16.3. The effects of dietary fructose and glucose, on insulin resistance and health.[127]

- Insulin resistance results from fructose and high fructose corn syrup (HFCS) in food and drinks

- Insulin resistance results from too many meals, particularly with carb snacking

- Environmental factors that cause cortisol to be increased including stress, poor sleep and lack of exercise

- High omega-6 to omega-3 ratios, which should be less than 4

- Smoking

So, anything that reduces the body's sensitivity to our own insulin is said to have increased insulin resistance. Increased insulin resistance is exactly the same as reduced insulin sensitivity. They both mean the same thing. This diagram outlines the effects of fructose on insulin resistance and health (figure 16.3). You can see how the blood sugar drops after a meal making

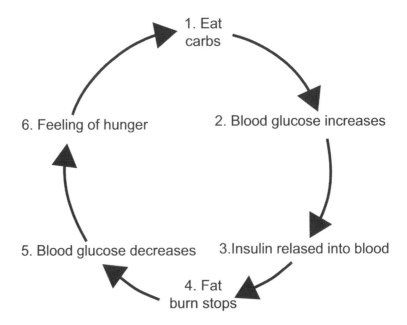

Figure 16.4. The refined and super-refined carbohydrate snacking-meal-snacking cycle of doom; turning off fat burning. The more time this happens the worse it gets, as insulin resistance builds and insulin circulates in the blood for a longer period.

us hungry again (figure 16.4) .

BASAL METABOLIC RATE

Our Basal Metabolic Rate (BMR) is the number of calories each of us requires to keep our body functioning for one day. Our BMR has developed with us for hundreds of generations as we have seen. One calorie is the energy required to heat 1 gram of water by 1 degree Celsius at 1 atmosphere pressure. One Kcal is the same for a kilogram of water.

Young men burn around 2000 calories per day, and this will happen quite effectively whether sleeping or watching the TV. It just happens, we burn our way through 2000 calories per day. And when we run for an hour, we burn an extra 500 calories. The furnace burns less in women and less in all of us as we age. In our body's furnace we burn our energy as follows; liver 25%, brain 20%, muscles 15%; kidneys 10%, heart 10% and the other 20% is spread amongst skin, gut, lungs and fat. Muscle is about three times as metabolically active as fat, pound for pound. But also note that muscle is a relatively small energy burner overall; so, don't fall prey to the "muscle burn your way to thinness" adverts. You can work out your BMR on the website.

Monique's sedentary BMR for one whole day is the equivalent of one burger, soda drink and fries at around 1100 calories. In energy terms, it is the same as running for two hours. That is the whole basis of a calorie-controlled diet, and we know that they fail in 19 out of 20 people when you observe them from long enough. Or as my friend says, "it's the low carb diet that works for me every time", without the slightest appreciation of his irony!

Start your calorie-controlled diet and weigh yourself in one year. Hey presto, you'll have put it all back on again; sound familiar? People go through this so many times, and we have seen the sarcopenic effects of yo-yo dieting in the food chapter. One of the commonest questions people ask me is why don't calorie-controlled diets work. The answer is hormonal homeostasis.

HOMEOSTASIS

Over those hundreds of generations, we can assume a few things. That our forefathers could fight and hunt on an empty belly. That is how our bodies have evolved. It is only very recently, that food became abundant; in fact, so much so that more people in our world die of overeating than under-nourishment.

And for hundreds of years we have desired the health and aesthetics of a lean and toned torso, both for ourselves and our breeding partners. And for young men, if they are to be successful and breed another generation, they should know that it is women who have the whip hand. Only half of all men on the planet will manage to breed. On average women will have two children and men one! Our ancestral family trees have more women than men by two to one. And apart from super-desirable men, who fall into a very small cohort, women almost always do the choosing.[10] So, the market for staying trim continues, even with modern dating and mobile phones; those pouting shots are much easier with a low level of body fat.

If you want a six-pack, you already have one, it's just covered by fat. If you think that the answer is sit-ups, then carry on. The way to a flat ripped abdomen is by fat loss not muscle gain. Well OK when your body fat is 13%, you can work on them and yes, they will get better. But, concentrate on the job at hand; if your body fat is 26% no matter how many years stubborn determination you show, we're never going to see them.

WHY CALORIE RESTRICTION FAILS AND FASTING WORKS

In extremis, calorie counting does work, but only for a short time. I'm not going to tell you that if I eat 20 burgers a day and you eat one lettuce leaf, that it won't make a difference; it will, obviously. But diets that make you calorie-count fail. That's not me saying that, it's scientific research.[126] There are two reasons, why calorie restrictive diets fail;

1. You've started a war with your body's hormones which is your survival system; your forefathers' best friend for millennia. Hormones, in your body will do everything in their power to keep you alive. And so, when you're in calorie deficit, they will slow down your metabolism, make you cold, tired and increase your appetite. And these powerful drivers will drive you mad; constantly craving food, agitated and tired. Your BMR will be reduced by your hormones. You will adjust to your new reduced calorie regimen, and you will stop losing weight.

2. These diets lower the calories by offering us hateful food that women, somehow tolerate for longer than men. Plates of rabbit food; lettuce, cress, celery and cucumber. Or even worse some hateful powdered mush, or a diet-bar filled with fructose. This can be maintained for a short while and then the desire for nutritious food kicks in. One day

you will crack and go off to the burger bar. And momentarily you will feel satiated.

Fasting is however a very different proposition to calorie restricting. By fasting, you are merely mimicking what our bodies have been accustomed to, since humans first stood upright; times of plenty and times of fasting. And, that doesn't create the upset in your hormones. In calorie restriction or small plates, or whatever fad-diet is currently fashionable, you are yelling at your hormones "I can beat you". And if you shout at your hormones, they'll win. They always do, which is why the odds for failure in any calorie restricted diet is 95% failures. Bad odds for you, but great odds for repeat business at the diet companies. Ca-Ching! Fasting is not accompanied by a reduction in BMR. The hormonal response to fasting is totally different to the response to calorie restriction. Our hormones make us perform well when we are fasting, but slow everything down when we are calorie restricting.

So, we whisper at our hormones, by mimicking scenarios our hormones are familiar with. Scenarios familiar to our hormones for generations. And guess what, they don't object and come happily on board. Learn to shed weight with your hormones on side, happy and contented.

MEAL FREQUENCY

We now know that 6 or more small meals, often recommended to newly diagnosed type 2 diabetics, and snacking, are associated with higher basal insulin levels, insulin resistance, metabolic syndrome and type 2 diabetes. The risks are discussed in the chapter on carbohydrates. Conversely, less frequent meals, at one, two or three per day, are also associated with many positive outcomes; increased insulin sensitivity, reduced hepatic fat concentration, weight loss, reduced inflammatory C-peptides, increased glucagon, and reduced fasting plasma glucose. So, we can very firmly say that less frequent meals and less snacking benefits our hormones and our long-term outlook. It allows us to switch on the fat burning again. Or for some people for the first time.

LEPTIN AND GHRELIN

Ghrelin is our hunger hormone and its release from the stomach wall causes hunger by affecting our brain. It is a powerful driver to eat more food and keep up our fat stores, for leaner times. It is increased by calorie restriction and is one of the factors that cause our calorie restrictive diets to fail. The longer the calorie restrictive diet, the higher the ghrelin. On the other hand, fasting does not increase ghrelin; in fact, fasting does quite the opposite and reduces ghrelin, hence no hunger.

Leptin is a very important hormone, produced by gut cells and fat cells. It works as our satiety hormone, telling us when we have had enough food. When blood sugar is high and insulin becomes resistant, their persistently high levels lead to leptin resistance. So, insulin resistance and leptin resistance go hand in hand. In these circumstances we have no satiety, to stop us eating. Importantly, high fructose corn syrup HFCS45 used in food and HFCS55 used in carbonated soft drinks cause leptin resistance directly. In time, this leads to cardiovascular disease, and obesity.[127]

CORTISOL

This is the fifth and last hormone you need to know about. We have introduced the two fat controllers, insulin and its opposite number glucagon. We've just met the hunger hormones leptin and ghrelin, that tell us whether we are full or hungry. And now one that may sound familiar. Cortisol is related to steroid creams you may have used for skin rashes or inhalers for asthma; these go by all sorts of proprietary names, but hydrocortisone or prednisolone have similar anti-inflammatory properties.

Cortisol is a glucocorticoid hormone; it affects the body widely and has receptors on many cells all over the body. It has an effect on our muscles, brains, lungs, heart and the rest of our hormonal or endocrine system. It also affects sugar metabolism. Cortisol is a steroid hormone primarily produced in the adrenal gland that sits on top of our two kidneys.

When you are escaping a loose tiger, you get what is called a "fight and flight" response from your central nervous system and your endocrine system. The hormones, adrenaline and cortisol are secreted. Your breath quickens, as does your heart rate; you can sense your heart pumping. There is a change to your muscle blood flow and you're very quickly readied for fight or flight. This is the essence of cortisol. It happens quickly, and when the threat goes, the cortisol returns to normal again over a matter of a few hours. The real problem with cortisol is when it doesn't return to normal but stays elevated for many hours, days or even long term. When we run a chronically elevated cortisol level in our blood, it is very bad for our health.[128] High cortisol is associated with;

- Shortened telomeres; chronic stress is the biggest association with shortened telomeres

- Increased obesity

- Increased visceral fat

- Increased midline subcutaneous fat, between the shoulder blades, over the back of the neck, face and stomach

- Insulin resistance and diabetes

- Digestive problems

- Muscle wasting and weakness

- The breakdown of muscle into glucose; gluconeogenesis

- Increased blood pressure

- Metabolic syndrome

- Poor sleep

- Cardiovascular disease; heart attacks and strokes

- Infections and immune system weakness

- Decreased libido; sexual drive

- Poor memory

- Poor cognitive ability

- Increased anxiety

- Reduced immune response and infections

- Raised eye pressure

- Glaucoma, a condition of raised pressure in the eye resulting in blindness if untreated

- The causes of chronically raised cortisol are;

- Medical conditions affecting the adrenal gland or pituitary gland at the base of the brain; Cushing's syndrome

- It can be caused by steroid medications taken orally or topically in the form of creams

- Estrogen elevation in females

- Stress and in particular how any individual responds to stress

The ways to reduce your lifestyle related raised cortisol are;

- Learn how to recognize when you are becoming stressed occurs

- Learn how to deal with your stress in a healthy way

- Regular sleep patterns and getting enough; 6-8 hours; 7 hours is the magic number

- Yoga and meditation

- Laughter and having fun with friends

- Spirituality

- Omega-3 fatty acids

- Good karma; try to be the best person and help others

- Healthy diet

- Your partner, caressing and caring for each other

- Stroking goes both ways for de-stressing you and your pet

In the wellness chapter we will look at the most important of these in more detail.

CHAPTER WHISPERINGS

- We've gone through two carbohydrate revolutions
- The second carbohydrate revolution was in the last 100 years
- The second carbohydrate revolution increased our refined carbohydrates 50-fold
- The second carbohydrate revolution is big corporates pushing carbs
- The second carbohydrate revolution has bamboozled our hormones
- Refined and super-refined carbohydrates are killing us
- Insulin causes carb and fat storage
- When insulin is in our blood, no fat can be metabolized, just more stored
- When glucagon is increased fat is burned
- Glucagon is released when healthy gaps occur between meals
- Snacking prevents fat burn, our natural way of coping between meals
- Insulin resistance occurs when blood glucose is too high for too long
- Ghrelin is the hormone that makes us hungry; its opposite number indicating satiety is leptin
- Leptin, our satiety hormone is made resistant by fructose and HFCS
- Ghrelin, our hunger hormone is designed for times when food is scarce, not plentiful
- Low meal frequency is critical for health
- BMR is basal metabolic rate
- Our hormones keep us alive; hormonal homeostasis
- Why calorie restrictive diets fail and get our hormones offside
- How fasting keeps our hormones quietly on-side and happy

- How cortisol is a short-term friend and a long-term enemy and how to reduce it

CHAPTER 17

HORMONES AND FASTING

"The philosophy of fasting calls upon us to know ourselves, to master ourselves, and to discipline ourselves the better to free ourselves. To fast is to identify our dependencies, and free ourselves from them"

Tariq Ramadan

INTRODUCTION

We have seen that fasting is completely different from calorie restricting, or calorie counting. To be perfectly clear, what we mean by fasting is variable intermittent fasting, and for simplicity called fasting from this point on. In this chapter, I shall explain why the ancient practice of fasting is a sensible addition to the diet-whisperer plan. In the 21st century, we have lost some of our vital links with religious fasting and our forefathers' healthy fasting habits. The result has been a generation of people who think fasting is uncomfortable, unnecessary and dangerous. It is not and they are very wrong. But such is this ingrained attitude, that I never tell people when I fast. I get bored explaining the benefits against the prejudices and ignorance of others.

Fasting is completely different from calorie restriction. A calorie restriction diet involves long-term reduction of calories by 20-40%. This can be achieved by changing the type of food eaten, reducing the amount of food eaten, or a combination of both. Importantly, the number of meals each day is either the same or increased. Intermittent or periodic fasting involves periods of 12 hours or more, when no food or drink is taken. Fasting periods are interspersed with meals that are not calorie restricted.

In calorie restriction, hormonal homeostasis slows the body down, reduces body temperature and reduces the energy consumption or BMR. Your hormones will perceive a threat of starvation and will act to conserve energy. Weight loss suddenly grinds to a halt. In fasting, your hormones react in a totally different way. Instead of shutting your body down, they allow repair and regeneration. Fasting increases your stress resistance, suppresses inflammation and improves blood glucose regulation. Fasting improves these health indicators, and they carry over into the fed state. This has the effect of improving mental and physical performance and increasing resistance to disease. Let's look at the 10 commonest misconceptions;

1. Three meals a day is best. Wrong, reducing EatSpan and lengthening FastSpan increase fat burn and weight loss.

2. Missing a meal puts the body into starvation mode. Wrong, unlike fasting, calorie restriction puts the body into starvation mode. And calorie restriction makes us cold, hungry, sleepy and miserable and turns down our metabolism. Fasting causes none of these symptoms.

3. Breakfast is the most important meal and gets your metabolism going. Wrong, breakfast breaks the benefits of the overnight fast. There is no evidence that it helps with fat burn. In fact, it turns the fat burn off, making us anabolic again. The more carbohydrates for breakfast, the more severe the insulin rise, the more severe the inhibition of fat burning. If you have to eat breakfast, at least go to work on an egg.

4. Eating small meals more frequently turns up the metabolism, thus burning more fat. Wrong, it increases insulin release and fat storage. It inhibits fat burning.

5. Fasting causes hunger. Wrong, fasting prevents hunger. Hunger gets worse with calorie restriction, multiple meals, and both refined and super-refined carbohydrates.

6. Fasting causes harm. Wrong, our bodies were designed to fast, and we survived intermittent fasting for 200,000 years. Fasting improves general health indicators, slowing and reversing aging and disease processes. It is known to promote mental and physical health and improve our spirituality. It is highly correlated with human wellness and longevity.

7. Fasting causes cell damage. Wrong, fasting is associated with healthy cell renewal, reduced aging and autophagy.

8. Fasting can harm our brain as our brain needs dietary carbohydrates. Wrong, our brains can survive happily on ketone bodies, produced during fasting.

9. Fasting will upset blood glucose. Wrong, insulin levels and insulin resistance are reduced, fat burning increased, with major improvements in blood glucose regulation.

10. Fasting damages cells and the brain. Wrong, studies show cell renewal and autophagy as well as possible protective measures in central nervous disorders like epilepsy and possibly dementia.

The beneficial effects of intermittent or periodic fasting are not limited to, but include;

- Reduced weight

- Reduced visceral fat

- Reduced insulin levels and insulin resistance [129]

- Reduction in all the features associated with metabolic syndrome including bad cholesterol

- Increased uric acid*

- Increased Human Growth Hormone (HGH or somatotropin).[130] It increases fat burn directly on fat cells

- Increased autophagy; renewing cellular organelles and inducing the anti-aging process in all cells including the brain

- Increased mitophagy, or mitochondrial renewal. Conversely, we know that heart mitophagy is reduced by diabetes and age

- Increased cognition and clarity of thought

- Improved short term memory

- Reduced free radicals, reducing oxidative stress

- Increased stress resistance at the cellular level

- Reduced inflammation in many long-term conditions, such as asthma [131]

- Reduced gut inflammation and increased motility

- Reduction in blood pressure

- Reduction in resting heart rate

- Reduction in C-reactive protein, a marker of inflammation

- Activation of sutuins, in a similar way to resveratrol, reducing oxidative stress and increasing mitophagy

- Increased gut microbiome diversity

- Fasting consistently increases lifespan in animals

- May have a role in cancer prevention, treatment and tumor suppression

- May have a role in delayed aging

We know that when we avoid refined carbohydrates, introduce intermittent fasting, reduce meal numbers, increase FastSpan and reduce EatSpan, we get positive effects on both our mental and physical health. We straighten out our hormones for wellness, longer healthspan and longer lifespan. We know that the induced autophagy is associated with reduced aging. And we are able to achieve permanent weight loss.

* Raised uric acid levels may have some anti-inflammatory effects.[132] It should be noted that gout may occur as uric acid goes up, and when it comes down. Uric acid directly competes for secretion in the urine in the kidney with ketone bodies. So, as ketone bodies increase, uric acid secretion reduces and blood uric acid rises. But in the fasted state in studies, gout did not occur.[133]

KETONE BODIES AS OUR FASTING FUEL

We know that there is no essential carbohydrate needed for our metabolism. We have already discussed why unrefined carbohydrate fiber is necessary to feed our gut microbiome and for gut health. It is true that our macronutrient metabolism can survive just fine without carbs. Yes, our red blood cells can only use glucose for metabolism. And our brain cannot use fats or proteins, as they cannot cross the blood brain barrier. It is true that 5-10% of our brain can only use glucose. But 90-95% of our brain can utilize either glucose or ketone bodies.

The ketone bodies, beta-hydroxybutyrate (BHB) and acetoacetate (AA), are produced from fats by the liver, when our glucose is in short supply, at the behest of our hormone glucagon. Our brain can not only survive on ketone bodies, but positively thrive. When metabolized for energy in our brain, they produce less oxidative stress than when we use glucose alone. So, when we switch to ketone bodies, we are helping to detox our brain. And low-carb diets, like keto, paleo and fasting, all create the right environment for ketone production, and for our brain to use them for metabolism. Research is ongoing on the role of ketones in the treatment of Parkinson's disease, epilepsy, dementia and other neurological conditions.

So, we have established that we need some carbohydrate, specifically glucose for part of our brains and all of our red blood cells. And we definitely need this to be available 24/7. But we do not need this glucose from food. Our hormonal homeostasis saves us yet again. When we fast or do not consume dietary carbs, our hormone glucagon kicks into action, and we start to live off the fat of the land. Or in this case, the fat of the liver and body. Our hormones keep our blood glucose within the normal range 24 hours a day. Instead of dietary glucose, we chop off glucose from our liver glycogen and send it into the blood. A process called glycogenolysis or "glycogen lysing; cutting the bonds". This lasts for 8-15 hours, until the 100 grams of stored liver glycogen is depleted. To prevent a fall in blood glucose at this point, is where things get interesting and a process of glucose production from non-carbohydrates commences. A bit like the sergeant calling his troops onto the parade ground in the early hours, there is a sudden awakening of these hormones in the liver, kidney and to a lesser extent in the bowel.

This process is called gluconeogenesis, or "glucose-new-creation". This process then maintains our blood glucose, by producing glucose from fats and proteins. Once again, we have shown that our brain and red blood cells can be maintained safely, by the upregulation of gluconeogenic hormones which upregulate the enzymes when needed. And no carbohydrates are required, dietary or stored. In a fasted state gluconeogenesis will happen on day two. On day three, our liver will begin to produce the ketone bodies. Our breath becomes "sickly sweet' with the smell of ketones, and we have reached a ketogenic state. In this state, our sugar requirements go down further as our brain shifts 90% of its metabolism to ketone bodies, with the antioxidant benefits mentioned above.

During intermittent fasting;

- We must maintain our blood glucose within strict levels every minute of every hour of every day for life, and we can do this without dietary carbohydrates

- Our brain and red blood cells initially use glucose from stored liver glycogen

- Our brain and red blood cells can later use glucose produced by gluconeogenesis, using fat and protein

- Eventually we reduce our brains energy requirement for glucose by 90%, as it switches to ketone bodies made in the liver from fats

TERMS USED IN FASTING METABOLISM

Metabolism, storage and production of glucose.

Glycolysis: Glucose to Pyruvate (Energy production)

Gluconeogenesis: Pyruvate to Glucose (Glucose from other macronutrients)

Glycogenesis: Glucose to Glycogen (storage)

Glycogenolysis: Glycogen to Glucose (breakdown)

HORMONAL CHANGES WITH FASTING

Effects of fasting

The first thing to say, as always, is discuss this with your doctor who will be able to support your plan to get lighter, fitter and healthier. Talking to your doctor is also a must if you are on any medications or have any co-existing diseases. For example, diabetes or hypertension may require a reduction or even a cessation in treatment, and it must be your doctor who guides you through this reduction in treatments. How exciting would that be!

First Four Hours

The macronutrients, fat, carbs and protein are broken down by digestion into their constituent parts, fatty acids, sugars, and amino acids and then absorbed from the small gut into the bloodstream. As we have seen all three macronutrients can, in turn, be stored as fat. When glucose is taken in excess of that required for immediate energy, and our glycogen levels are full, the excess blood glucose will be stored as fat. Insulin will mediate this. Insulin also mediates the building of muscle; again, any spare amino acids will also be stored as fat. So, our normal fed state is one of circulating insulin, with glycogen stores fully replenished. Our insulin peaks and then fades back down.

Our glucose is now stored away, and the circulating blood glucose falls into the normal range. Note that when refined carbs are eaten, the blood glucose falls before the insulin has stopped circulating. This overshoot can cause a period of relatively low blood sugar, making us hungry and angry. The word "hangry" combines them both, explaining the peak in road rage at 6 o'clock in the evening (figure 17.1).

When the blood sugar drops, and our insulin finally washes out, the body's constant need for sugar remains. Without more food the circulating blood glucose gets slowly used up. But, should this go on, the blood glucose would fall to dangerously low levels. To prevent this, glucagon hormones from the pancreas are released increasing the blood glucose.

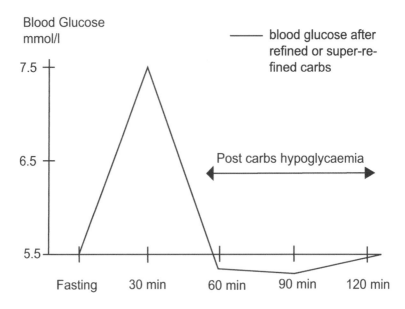

Figure 17.1. Spike in blood sugar following refined or super-refined carbohydrates. The remaining blood insulin pushes down the blood glucose, making us hungry and angry, or "hangry".

4-11 Hours

Here we go from the storage of glucose (insulin-mediated), to glycogen breakdown (glucagon-mediated). This maintains our blood glucose in spite of the glucose "pull" from our red blood cells and brain. At only 2% of our body mass, our brain uses 20% of the body's daily energy burn. That is 400 calories, equating to our whole glycogen liver stores of 100 grams. Note, the 300 grams of glycogen stored in skeletal muscle is not available for this purpose and continues to be available for locomotion. It also represents our natural fast from supper to breakfast. So, glucagon keeps our blood sugar ticking along from our glycogen stores. It also is able to top up this process by gluconeogenesis; creating glucose for our bloodstream from fats and amino acids. Most cells can use fats and proteins for energy directly; the brain and red blood cells are exceptions. Thanks to glucagon, it looks after matters for us. If at this stage, we take food the cycle starts all over again. If we continue to fast, then;

After 12-48 hours

The glycogen stores are depleted, and our hormones now switch us into full ketogenesis. That means, "ketone-making". The ketone bodies produced are acetone, acetoacetate and beta-hydroxybutyrate. The brain now switches to 70% ketone use for its energy. So, the brain uses 280 calories from ketone bodies AA and BHB which can unlike other macronutrients cross the blood-brain-barrier. Simultaneously, gluconeogenesis continues producing new glucose from fats and muscle, as required. This can trickle out 80-100 grams of glucose per day into our blood equating to 320-400 calories. Our hormones have changed our metabolism to protect us with at least 200-400 calories to spare of glucose. And it did this without any requirement for dietary macronutrients of any type. Interestingly there is less oxidative stress around when our brain is 70% powered on ketones bodies. It is thought this may offer some protection for diseases such as epilepsy, Parkinson's and dementia. It is somewhat perplexing to imagine such potential benefits from fasting. Our body maintains a beautiful balance though hormonal homeostasis. It's how we've lived for 200,000 years and our genes have encoded us with the ability to fast and thrive. Fasting is a time for repair and regeneration, followed by feasting, where we have building and growth.

After 2-5 days of fasting

Circulating insulin deceases significantly by 20-30% and ghrelin (our hunger hormone) decreases, day-on-day resulting in much less hunger. Repeated fasting will not only reduce insulin resistance, but also your chance of developing metabolic syndrome and type 2 diabetes. At the same time, there is a reduction in insulin resistance and leptin resistance. Autophagy will increase, replenishing our cells and making our gut and skin healthier. Our immune system cells are renewed. Autophagy is associated with slowed aging. This may, particularly in men, produce skin shrinkage as the weight comes off.[123]

Your Whispering Regimen

Diet-whispering is not only about whispering to your hormones, but is about self-empowerment, putting you back in charge. It's about quick results and sustainability. It allows you to have the skills you need to keep your hormones working with you, helping you achieve your weight goals. No longer will your hormones be in charge of your fat stores. You will be in control of your fat stores, so you can target your weight, get there and stay there. If you are like me, at times you will err with food and drink. That does not matter. To err is human; as is enjoying family, friends and life. What matters is that you will be able use your hormones to regain control quickly. You will see quick results, not just today, but forever. To use my skiing-diet metaphor, you can plan to go off-piste without fear, in the knowledge that you have the skills to get back. At that point, you really are in charge of your nutrition and weight; your hormones helping you rather than hindering you. You will have learned the trusted ways your ancestors lived in harmony with their hormones.

Once you have completed the whisperer-loss 12-week plan, you will be in control and able to form your own regimen. Alternate day fasts, one or two meals per day, or three or four-day fasts once a fortnight. There is no right, nor wrong. You can see what suits you. I know on my three-day fasts that I feel great on day two and better on day three. Not hungry at all, clear of mind and really fresh. What we know, is there will be a combination from this book that will suit you, and you will come to love. And your new waistline may please you too! There's always pleasure in buying a pair of smaller jeans. Oh, the joys of being a whisperer!

SUPPLEMENTS

When Monique and I fast, we do not take anything but water, black tea or coffee, and ensure that 3 liters minimum fluids, is taken each 24 hours. I tend to monitor my intake by thirst and ensuring my urine is no darker than a light straw color. Darker means possible dehydration. If this happens, drink more and it will lighten. We do not use supplements during fasting, as these may increase insulin and break the fast. However, we do use the following supplements, at the end of each fasting period.

- Multivitamins

- Cod liver oil

- Calcium

- Vitamin D

CHAPTER WHISPERINGS

- Fasting is an ancient practice; we have lost connection with the fasting our forefathers practiced

- Fasting is not dangerous

- Fasting is associated with positive changes in our brains

- Fasting improves health markers

- Fasting improves cellular health and turnover, or autophagy

- Fasting benefits the gut microbiome

- Unrefined carbohydrates are essential for our microbiome

- All three macronutrients can produce glucose to protect our red blood cells and brain

- Our brain can survive on ketone bodies and less than 20% glucose

- We do not need any refined or super-refined carbohydrates in our diet and should be discarded except for rare treats

- With 3 liters per day of fluids we can fast safely for days or weeks. Build up slowly

- Fasting should come after you have become fat adapted, as explained in the next two chapters

- Supplements may be helpful as outlined above

CHAPTER 18

PHILOSOPHY AND FASTING

"Where there is distress that cannot be removed, my religion teaches me to fast and pray"

M. Gandhi

INTRODUCTION

We know fasting is a powerful tool for burning fat; very powerful. And fasting ranges from skipping breakfast to missing food safely for days on end. But before we fast, we must fat adapt. Fat adaptation allows our bodies faster and better access our fat stores, when food is scarce, as you will see in the next chapter. These two are practiced sequentially; only fast when you have successfully fat adapted.

Combining these, we get extremely powerful fat loss. And we gain consent from our own hormones and our bodies are able to slip seamlessly into periods of fasting. Then, when fasting and fat adaptation are combined, your hormones will come into balance and you will regain complete control of your weight.

All major religions practice fasting, and longer periods of fasting lead to clarity of mind and even spirituality for some. Our recent dietary switch from fats, proteins and unrefined carbohydrates, to a more refined carbohydrates is killing us. It is making us ill and obese. It is making our hormones anabolic and preventing the normal metabolism that gave our ancestors a sufficient advantage to pass on their genes. And the food laboratories of corporates are keeping us snacking and keeping us ill.

I question myself, whenever I eat a burger. How good did it taste, and how did I feel for the following few hours? The answer to the taste was of course great. That's why the corporates spend millions hitting that "bliss-point". And the answer to how I felt afterwards was, tired, bloated and frankly very stodgy. A few hours later and I'm hungry again. And my third question is, was it worth it? The answer to this has become more strongly "no" the older and wiser I get.

When you have the ability to fast properly, you notice that hunger fades every hour and every day. And your mind clears of all the noise and mayhem; then you see the amazing benefits of fasting, on your body and your mind.

RELIGION, EQUALITY AND FASTING

In the UK and US, we have the good fortune of living in free democratic societies, and mainly thanks to our forefather's faith in Judaism and Christianity. Douglas Murray in his book, The Strange Death of Europe, believes our future will to some extent be determined by the treatment of our churches.[134] Murray, an atheist, believes that Christianity is central to everything we have. I believe that the good in believing, lies in the believing as well as the belief per se. Everywhere we turn to in the UK and the US, we see the products of our ancestors' belief in God. If we look around, we see that our lives are interlaced with the results of Christianity. Hospitals, schools, architecture, classical music, fine arts, the great universities, human rights, workers' rights; the list goes on. We have been exceptionally lucky.

Christianity created a hub, a network and a community. Community correlates powerfully with human longevity in the world's Blue Zones. Our religious community provided us with rules and a moral compass. Are we coping well without this community? And when it comes to eating and drinking, have we lost self-control and self-respect? We care less about what we eat, how we eat or how indeed how we look. If you question the latter, google 1950s images. When times get tough, do we get our comfort from food rather than community and spirituality? Even the less spiritual amongst us can see the values that spirituality brings. Perhaps Nietzsche was right, "God is dead". Will we see a resurgence or even a non-believing Christianity? I suspect not, but time will tell.

There is no proof that there is a causal relationship between the vertiginous fall in Christian worship and the rise in obesity, but there is correlation. We know that obesity has not one single causative factor, nor one single cure. But it is an interesting thought about our spiritual affairs in general, not just related to obesity.

It is also interesting to note that in all major faiths, fasting has played its part for eons. For Jews, a 25-hour fast for Yom Kippur. In Christianity, Jesus fasted for 40 days and 40 nights, as part of his spiritual preparation, which is now observed during Lent. Roman Catholics refrain from meat on Fridays and remember the life of Jesus and the Virgin Mary. They also practice sobriety, contemplation and abstinence.

In the Old Testament, from some 700 BC, The Book of Isaiah;

> "Shout it aloud, do not hold back. Raise your voice like a trumpet. Declare to my people their rebellion and to the descendants of Jacob their sins. For day after day they seek me out; they seem eager to know my ways, as if they were a nation that does what is right and has not forsaken the commands of its God. They ask me for just decisions and seem eager for God to come near them. 'Why have we fasted,' they say, 'and you have not seen it? Why have we humbled ourselves, and you have not noticed?'

> Yet on the day of your fasting, you do as you please and exploit all your workers. Your fasting ends in quarreling and strife, and in striking each other with wicked fists. You cannot fast as you do today and expect your voice to be heard on high.

> Is this the kind of fast I have chosen, only a day for people to humble themselves? Is it only for bowing one's head like a reed and for lying in sackcloth and ashes? Is that what you call a fast, a day acceptable to the Lord?

> Is not this the kind of fasting I have chosen: to lose the chains of injustice and untie the cords of the yoke, to set the oppressed free and break every yoke? Is it not to share your food with the hungry and to provide the poor wanderer with shelter-- when you see the

naked, to clothe them, and not to turn away from your own flesh and blood? Then your light will break forth like the dawn, and your healing will quickly appear; then your righteousness will go before you, and the glory of the Lord will be your rear guard. Then you will call, and the Lord will answer; you will cry for help, and he will say: Here am I.

If you do away with the yoke of oppression, with the pointing finger and malicious talk, and if you spend yourselves in behalf of the hungry and satisfy the needs of the oppressed, then your light will rise in the darkness, and your night will become like the noonday. The Lord will guide you always; he will satisfy your needs in a sun-scorched land and will strengthen your frame. You will be like a well-watered garden, like a spring whose waters never fail. Your people will rebuild the ancient ruins and will raise up the age-old foundations; you will be called Repairer of Broken Walls, Restorer of Streets with Dwellings.

If you keep your feet from breaking the Sabbath and from doing as you please on my holy day, if you call the Sabbath a delight and the Lord's holy day honorable, and if you honor it by not going your own way and not doing as you please or speaking idle words, then you will find your joy in the Lord, and I will cause you to ride in triumph on the heights of the land and to feast on the inheritance of your father Jacob. For the mouth of the Lord has spoken."

In Buddhism, monks fast from lunchtime through to breakfast, whilst followers practice mindful eating; touch each pistachio nut, look at it in your hand, smell it, imagine where and how it was grown, then eat each one slowly, realizing its true pleasure. The antithesis is eating in front of the television, when we may reasonably ask, how many did pistachios do we remember eating?

Ramadan, the ninth month of the Islamic calendar, when God revealed the first verses of the Quran to Mohammed, is when Muslims fast from dawn till dusk. The meal that follows is a joyous time for family, friends and togetherness.

In Hinduism, coinciding with phases of the moon, Ekadashi is practiced twice monthly and worshiping the God Gamesh, spiritual contemplation and fasting are often observed. Arguably the most famous Hindu, Mahatma Gandhi, said, "where there is distress that cannot be moved, my religion teaches me to fast and pray". And to be fair, he was pretty well and fit for his three score years and ten. His fasting was, however, unable to save him from the Beretta's three bullets fired at close range. Gandhi also said, "my idea of society is that we are all born equal, meaning we have the right to equality of opportunity, but we do not share the same capacity". Gandhi practiced and prescribed self-control through spirituality and fasting. His individuality should be seriously considered by us all, particularly when we consider spirituality, fasting and eating. Plough your own furrow and ignore the group mentality dictating three meals a day and the commercially driven lunacy of snacking. Whilst there may be abundant corporate sugar-polluting foods confusing our hormones and influencing our choices, we must not become the victim that "equality of outcome" preaches. It is down to us, to show some discipline and some backbone and learn from the past. With knowledge, we can master our strong hormonal drives, and once again take control of our destiny.

PHILOSOPHY, SPIRITUALITY AND FASTING

The whole subject of philosophy, spirituality and fasting is fascinating, and about which much has been written across the centuries.

One common theme is that finding your own spirituality is undoubtedly empowering and enriching. Those who find they can reach out from the earth, to the sky and the stars above, can break their earthly shackles, and rejoice in living on a higher plane. Should this be your want, fasting will help you achieve this. It will also diminish your desire for more refined and fancy foods. Your palate is cleansed and the yearning for those sugary-delights wanes. Fried foods, stuffed with omega-6s, once favorites, take on a new and sickly demeanor. Even your natural desire for less virtuous pastimes, fades in an inexplicable manner.

When you have the chance to fast for longer than one day, you have the chance to reconnect with your soul. Be thoughtful, contemplative and reflect. Dream and watch clouds or meditate, relax and reconnect with your soul. Scribble, draw or write. Or do nothing at all; and allow others this courtesy too. Learn once again to switch off.

There is much more to fasting than you can imagine, right up to the moment you yourself achieve it. The cleansing of body and mind is truly beautiful. Of course, there will be hiccups, headaches, shakes and migraines, but they soon pass. Like all changes, it takes time to learn the nuances.

Fasting is as old as the hills. In the West, our bodies are carbohydrate addicted. We are also fat fuel inhibited. This makes fasting much more difficult, so firstly we must fat adapt our bodies. This will allow us to access the pleasures and other benefits from fasting. Another factor in your success, is that unless you live alone, you will never achieve this without your family's support. If necessary, take yourself off in the campervan to the hills or a lake, or to a silent retreat, or better still a silent fasting retreat. And, find the purity of a few days or a week fasting, drinking just water and black tea or coffee. Reconnect yourself with nature.

Plato said that he fasted for greater mental and physical efficiency. Hippocrates and Paracelsus, both advocated fasting. With the former saying that "everyone has their own physician inside them" and "that to eat when ill is to feed the sickness". Plutarch a middle Platonist philosopher said, "instead of using medicine, fast a day". Wise words.

EATING HABITS

In England, table manners were an intrinsic part of the very essence of being English, declining in the latter part of the last century. It took my parents decades before spaghetti was allowed at supper. Also, turning the spaghetti in a spoon, let alone with the fork in the right hand was regarded as a capital offense; etiquette dictated we should use the side of the plate. To this day, I baulk at the very offering of a spoon with spaghetti. When we eat with our families properly, we can concentrate on the food we eat, respect its source and be thankful that we have food in abundance. We get joyous family time by this practice. And, in our house mobile phones are not allowed at mealtimes.

Communal eating, which I adore, with copious French claret, is a time to eat, drink and be merry. It's not a time for restraint or picky dieting. Remember, picky eaters at a party, soon become one of the 5% of people in the world describing themselves as unhappily alone. Food, friends and family should be enjoyed. Meals bring people together and a few rules can help.

The next time you eat, tray on lap watching the television, see if you can remember eating your food and how much was eaten; I certainly can't.

THREE MEALS A DAY: NONSENSE

So, communal eating is terrific fun, but it has its drawbacks. Firstly, it should be amongst things we do some of the time. The exception not the rule. The rigid three meals a day began a few hundred years ago. A great idea, but only if you're laboring all day. In the middle of the 20th century, even those that labored were gradually being assisted by mechanization. The Irish immigrant trench diggers in the UK, were wiry with massive strong hands covered in asbestos-like skin. Those men's children now operate excavators, but still consume the same food and of course their beloved stout. They are more obese than their fathers. So, there was a role for three meals a day, in agrarian and industrial laboring communities, but now in the post-industrial age, it's time for a rethink.

The Romans ate only one meal a day at lunchtime. In post-war England, breakfast was promoted as the most important meal of the day. The vast majority of adults just do not need three meals. And if like me, you've struggled with your weight, that means you and me too.

We need to control the madness of three meals a day. But when you do eat your meals, make it a rejoiceful one with your family at the end of the day. No phones at the table, no radio or TV, just celebrating the food and the family. Talking, rejoicing and being happy. Seek out your individualism and develop your spirituality along with your weight loss.

WARNING

Firstly, when you are fasting, be careful who you tell. It becomes very boring when people tell you it's dangerous! If you are able to enrich your whole life with fasting, you may start to find the eating habits of those around you gluttonous and disgusting. You have been warned. So, as I said above, get your partner to come on the journey with you. Neither of you will regret it. Fasting and fat adapting are difficult at first, but when you get it right and learn the benefits, I suspect you like me, will never eat three meals in a day again.

CHAPTER WHISPERINGS

- Fasting is as old as the hills and is safe
- Fasting is practiced in all major religions
- Fasting, spirituality and well-being are all connected
- People are addicted to carbohydrate, sugar and flour rich foods
- Fasting is made very difficult and miserable by carbohydrate addiction
- We need to fat adapt before we try fasting, so our body can use fat as our fuel
- Fat adaptation, not only allows our body access to fat stores, but makes fasting easier
- As eating habits have changed, so has our ability to contemplate what and how much food we consume
- Eating three meals a day is only 200 years old; fine when work was physically hard, but in our modern world has gone way past its sell by date

CHAPTER 19

FAT ADAPTATION

"There is only one way to survive and thrive when faced with circumstances out of our control: ADAPT"

Charles F Glassman

INTRODUCTION

Like Glassman, we face circumstances where our metabolism is out of our control. And fat adaptation is the process by which we change the body from carbohydrate burning to fat burning.

During the coronavirus lockdown, I tried to buy some natural yogurt in my local supermarket. The dairy shelves were bare, except for full fat yogurt. All the low-fat yogurts had gone. Imagine all the fat people clambering to buy their beloved low-fat foods, thinking that these will help with their diet. The beauty of a high-fat meal is the small rise in insulin, compared with carbs and proteins. Therefore, there is reduced fat storage and a quick return to burning fat as our fuel. In low-fat yogurt, when the fat is replaced by carbohydrates, the insulin release is greater, preventing us from switching on our fat burning. This has the added downside of making us hungry again. Once again low-fat food exposes our ignorance.

The calorie value of fats is 9 calories per gram and sugar and protein are both 4 calories per gram. So, if you eat more fat, you get more calories; true, but that is just looking the wrong way through the telescope. Look at it the other way around. We want to reduce our fat stores, by using it to create our body's energy. As it is calorie dense, we can utilize it as a source of power; it's a highly efficient fuel source. In the previous chapter, we learned how fat was a huge store of energy for athletes running very long distances. Here we see how fat is also an abundant fuel for everyone else going about their normal daily routines. But first we need to learn to switch on fat burning.

We know that calories in, does not equal calories out, because of the effects of different macronutrients on our hormones, particularly insulin. From the chart we can see that fat has a very much smaller insulin response compared with carbohydrates, with protein between the two (Figure 15.3). Ideally, we want a small insulin response; that is the area under the line on the graph to be small and short, so we can return to fat burning. It should be noted that insulin and glucose hanging around in the blood two hours after food are predictors of early death.[24]

Hunger is driven by eating carbs; increasing with the frequency and the refinement of the carbs. So, our feeling of hunger is always, and I repeat always, caused by the hormonal effect of the last snack or meal. If this describes you then you may have;

FAT FUEL INHIBITION (FFI)

This is our body's inability to switch from carbs onto fat for fuel. We have effectively made ourselves addicted to the short-term rush of refined and super-refined carbohydrates. A cycle repeated over and over during the day and sometimes night. Check if you recognize any of these symptoms;

- Food does not fill you up, or give you a feeling of satiety

- After meals, you often feel tired

- You get low energy periods during your day, particularly after lunch

- You desire a siesta in the afternoon

- You lose weight for a period of time, only to put it back on

- You have mood swings during the day, particularly irritability

- You are often hungry, and snacking brings relief

- When hungry, you get shakes, and or get sweaty

- When hungry, you get headaches or migraines

- You find it hard to sleep on an empty stomach

- You wake during the night feeling hungry

- A snack makes you feel normal again

- You get brain fog if you don't snack

- You tend to eat carbs for snacks; pastries, cake, muffins, cookies, candy bars

- You drink soda drinks to satisfy your hunger symptoms

If you suffer just one of these, you may well have fat fuel inhibition. The great news is that with a little help we can turn this around and put you back in control.

LEXUS HYBRID AND YOU

A while back, we bought a Lexus 4x4; a well-known hybrid. Not for any ecological reasons, but because I was fascinated by the idea of a seamless switching from between its two fuel sources, gasoline and electricity. It was a very good, reliable car and yes, it switched absolutely seamlessly between fuel sources.

Our body can fuel itself through carbohydrates, fats or protein. Since our ancestors escaped the saber-toothed tigers and would walk and run miles to get food, generally it is accepted that muscle is not only useful, but necessary for survival. Accordingly, muscle protein is spared as a fuel under most circumstances and preserved until last. That leaves us with our two main fuels, carbohydrates and fat. It can also be safely assumed that our ancestors could do all that was required for survival on an empty stomach. They were constantly fat adapted, as they had no refined or super-refined carbs to munch on, as they hunted or evaded the tiger. Darwin taught us, the genes from the losers didn't get passed on.

So, like the Lexus, we also have two energy systems. The first, is the carbohydrate burning system and the second the fat burning system. Like the Lexus, we can also switch seamlessly from one to the other. The choice of fuel the Lexus uses, is controlled by a microchip. The fuel we use is controlled by our hormones. So, if you live on a diet of refined and super-refined carbohydrates, your hormones will store these carbs as glycogen and fat. Carbohydrate food raises your insulin the highest and the longest. If you eat refined carbohydrates every few hours (remember that biscuit with your coffee), your hormone insulin will be constantly raised. And, when you have insulin circulating, your body is unable to use fat as a fuel. You are in a carbohydrate-only fuel state. And, to make it worse, you will be converting excess carbs into stored fat. Let us look at our two fuel reserves (figure 19.1).

Firstly, carbohydrates are re-strung and stored in the liver and muscles as glycogen. Glycogen is very rapidly available to produce our energy ATP tokens, with or without oxygen. Carbs can produce ATP instantly, and is used by our muscles when we begin to move. In the liver, glycogen is broken down to maintain the baseline blood glucose levels, by glycogenolysis. We have a limited store of glycogen, at around 400g or 1600 calories. Glycogen will last us for about 14-16 hours of fasting or 60-120 minutes of vigorous exercise. But, fear not, when the glycogen is depleted, our bodies can manufacture glucose from fats, by gluconeogenesis.

Secondly, fats. These can also be used as our energy source. And unlike the carbs, we have 135,000 calories in our 15 kg of stored fat (figure 19.2). Triglycerides, our stored fats, are broken down with 95% of the energy coming from the fatty acid chain components. As they are oxidized, they also produce ATP. This fat oxidation is a slower process and roughly speaking we get 20% more energy from carbohydrates than we do from fats per liter of oxygen inhaled. Give our hormones a free choice and they'll take the carbs, as the fast and easy option. And when we set up this cycle of eat carbs, snack carbs, feel hungry, snack carbs, carb lunch, feel hungry, snack carbs, there is no good reason for our hormones to change.

Our bodies are very adaptive; that is, they get used to the change. If you don't believe me think about walking or jogging. If you do it correctly

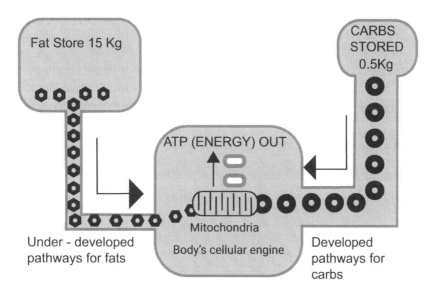

Figure 19.1. Dual fuel, cellular power in the human body. Notice the narrower access from the fat stores. Fat adaptation improves the access.

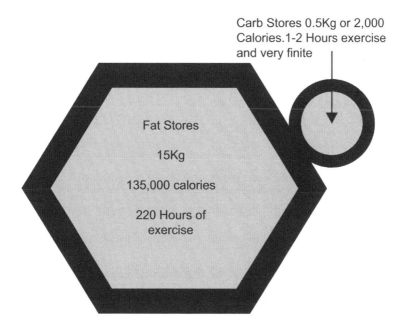

Figure 19.2 . Relative amounts of fat stored and carbohydrate stored in the human body.

your body soon adapts, and you find it easier. This is adaptation. As we humans increased the carbs in our diet, we went from being fat adapted to carb adapted. Even worse, our enzymes for fat burning became fewer and weaker. So, when we try to burn fat, we find we are fat fuel inhibited. When we first try, it's what makes us feel terrible. We need to build up these enzymes and pathways, so we are just as comfortable on either fuel. Now that Monique and I are fat adapted, it is by far my favorite state. We feel well and generally so much healthier and clearer of mind.

FAT ADAPTATION

Fat adaption is the first secret to ridding ourselves of excess fat. For the past 100 years we have fed on too much refined carbohydrate, at too high a frequency; think snacks. We have now learned that our fat burning is switched off by refined carbohydrates, and snacking. And the more months and years we do this, the more reliant we become on glucose as our fuel.

Whenever we run our carbohydrate stores down, we start to feel trembly and weak. We get the symptoms outlined above for carbohydrate addiction. The very moment we are about to switch our engine from carb-burning to fat-burning, we prevent this by having a cup of tea, or a biscuit. Or a slice of toast, or cake. We do this all day, every day. These habits keep us carbohydrate reliant and addicted. These bad teachings have made us into carbohydrate lemmings, heading for the vertiginous cliff that is metabolic disease. At some point we have to bite the bullet. We have to detox our body from carbohydrate addiction. We have to go cold turkey on the carbs.

It took Lexus millions of development hours and millions of development yen, to develop their hybrid. And, God gave us our hybrid system for free. Passed down successfully for generations from our hunter-gatherer forefathers, who used it day after day to hunt on an empty belly. We have stopped using our fat and the enzymes required for fat metabolism are depleted. Our highly refined carbohydrate diets have adapted us away from fat metabolism. And now we must learn to go back, losing our fat and making ourselves well again. Freeing ourselves from the clutch of the Grim Reaper, that is obesity and metabolic syndrome. We can simply learn to switch on the second of the two fuels we have powering us; our fat burning engine. Every time we eat refined carbohydrates as a meal or a snack, we turn off our fat burning engine. And the more frequent the meals and the higher and more refined the carbs, the more we suppress our fat burning engine.

It is very strange that the culture behind hybrid cars is to save the planet and everyone else, but we won't buy into saving ourselves. Corporatism is telling you to eat more food, more refined and more often. Just empower yourself, by doing the opposite. It is difficult for a week or two, but when you get there, it will be worth it. You will not even imagine how this will change your physical and mental well-being. And as many of my patients tell me, their lives are now filled with joy and spirituality. Joy that had long since been subsumed under the blanket of refined carbohydrate human misery. Fat adaptation puts you back in control of your weight and your well-being, both physical and mental.

FAT ADAPTATION IN TWO PHASES

There is nothing really complicated about fat adaptation, when you understand the basics. What you mustn't do is confuse uncomplicated with easy. I can tell you honestly, I found it pretty rough! Really rough for the first week, quite rough for the second and then saw light at the end of the tunnel by week 4. I really started to feel better by weeks 7 and 8 and had the benefit of having lost nearly 10 kg by this stage. It was quite remarkable. It is quite simply the best thing I have ever done for myself and Monique feels exactly the same. But ask your loved ones to support you as you get irritable and irrational. Some people get flu like symptoms. Some stomach upsets, others brain fog and sleepiness. It will be worth it. And if you fail, dust yourself down and start over. As coach John Wooden would say, "when you wake up make this day your masterpiece".[135]

The time period involved is highly individual, but the first phase will take between 2 and 4 weeks. It really does vary widely. It is very dependent on your current lifestyle, dietary habits and current fitness.

The human body adapts very well to change, so we help it back to its natural state, burning fats easily. The fat adaptation happens in two distinct phases; Phase 1, the high fat diet, and phase 2, high fat plus increasing FastSpan and Reducing EatSpan. If you are a bacon and egg sort of person, or a steak eater, we suggest you stay on those animal fats to begin with. Eventually we advise that you start to replace them with healthier fats, but not at the beginning, as there will be too many changes. If you're on a Mediterranean diet high in MUFAs and PUFAs, even better; stick with those.

Fat adaptation Phase 1;

- Start by adopting a ketogenic diet, with a maximum of 25-50 grams of carbs each day

- Fat will be 65%, proteins 35% and carbohydrates 5%

- You can calculate macronutrients in grams on the website

- Eat three meals per day and never snack in between

- Be prepared for the symptoms of "keto flu" as your body initially struggles without the refined carbohydrate "hits"; you are effectively going cold turkey on your refined carbs

- Stick with it because only when you have detoxed your carbs will your hormones be back in regular working order. In an emergency eat an apple, but better still try to ride the storm

- Talk to your family and tell them what you are doing because at times you will be irritable and difficult

- Don't weaken and have that carb hit. You need real strength in the first few weeks

- You can use any of the thousands of keto diets on the internet

- Do not snack between meals,

- Do not snack after your last meal in the evening, and breakfast the following day

- Continue with phase 1 until you have 4 weeks under your shrinking belt

Fat Adaptation Phase 2;

- On your second 4 weeks the food is the same, but here we start to increase the FastSpan and reduce the EatSpan

- So, on days off work, we suggest you take breakfast later

- Try combining it with lunch or brunch

- If you feel after a while you can skip breakfast, then do and have a two-meal day. You are a winner.

- Stick to trying to eat brunch later and your evening meal earlier

- Eating your evening meal just one hour earlier increases your overnight FastSpan significantly

- This all helps with your fat adaptation

- Eventually you will combine breakfast with lunch. Why not just eat your bacon and eggs for lunch?

At this stage you will be fat adapted, and you will no longer have those horrible symptoms of fat fuel inhibition. Your hormones and enzyme are now recovering back to their normal state.

FAT ADAPTATION AT THE CELLULAR LEVEL

Mitochondria are our cellular power stations. These tiny organelles lying in the body of our cells, or cytoplasm, produce our ATP energy tokens from oxidative metabolism. They do so from fats or carbs. When we fat adapt over time on a low-carbohydrate or fasting regimen our cells undergo some changes. And fastest of all when we do both.

Like all organelles, our mitochondria naturally become old and are continually replaced. This process in cells is known as autophagy, or specifically for mitochondria, mitophagy. This replacement cycle depends on your age, your genes, your fitness and how much exercise you take. For some people, their mitochondria will become fat adapted in 2-4 weeks, whilst in others it may take several months for all tissues to get fully fat adapted. Fat adaptation increases the size, turnover, efficiency and number of mitochondria. When you are fully fat adapted, your mitochondria in all cells will be happy burning fats as well as carbs. Your hormones will be better balanced, and you will be feeling on top of your health.

Fat adaptation is a state in your body when your mitochondria in every cell utilizes fats for fuel as their primary source of energy. Your insulin is raised less and less frequently. Your body can break down fat for fuel. Your brain will also be adapted to life on 70% ketone bodies. Your body and brain are now fully adapted to your new low-carb diet, fasting and cessation of snacking. Ketone measurements can at best be confusing. They may be useful when you start out to tell you when you are in a ketotic state. And by definition you will have to remain ketotic for fat adaptation to occur. There is no magical test to tell you when you have started to fat adapt or when it is completed. But you will have the following useful signs that you are fat adapted.

SIGNS OF FAT ADAPTATION

- Your brain will be clear, cognition and memory improved

- Hunger will have disappeared or be very much reduced

- After a meal you will feel full and satiated

- You will no longer suffer carbohydrate and junk food cravings

- You will lose that tired feeling after lunch

- You will have increased exercise endurance

- You will have increased energy levels

- You blood pressure will be lower

- Your resting heart rate will be lower

- You will sleep better, deeper and longer

- You will be less prone to dependent edema

- You will be burning fat and losing fat

ALCOHOL

For most people, we advise no alcohol during the first 8 weeks of the program. But that can be a bridge too far for some. So, we have some general advice. Try to drink alcohol that is low in carbs and only in the evening. Or lunchtime, if that is your routine. Alcohol is a toxin and so your liver will deal with this as a priority and forget about the fat burning. Even so, we are realists and if you do drink, we suggest the following in order of preference.

- Vodka with ice and a slice mixed with zero calorie sparkling water

- Gin with ice and a slice mixed with zero calorie sparkling water

- Gin or vodka with low-calorie, or zero calorie tonic

- Gin or vodka with naturally low-calorie tonic, but watch the carbs

- Red wine

- Dry white wine

- Champagne

- A splash of bitters can be welcome

- A slice of lime or lemon can be welcome

- Any high alcohol content shorts are OK too

Warnings.

Alcohol will slow down your fat adaptation and make it more difficult. Alcohol will be much more potent during and after fat adaptation, so your tolerance will be way down. And, you will be prone to very uncomfortable hypos the day after drinking, particularly after heavy sessions, often leading to high carb intake.

CHAPTER WHISPERINGS

- Fat burning is prevented in the presence of insulin

- Food, by stimulating insulin secretion, prevents fat burning

- The degree to which food turns off fat burning is related to the amount of insulin it produces

- Low-fat foods, that are carbohydrate enriched, elevate insulin

- Humans have a dual fuel system; we can fuel using either fats or carbohydrates

- Muscle protein is generally not used for fueling because of its importance

- Carbohydrate diets, in particular those with refined and super-refined carbohydrates switch off fat burning as a fuel

- Eating carbohydrates, not fat is what makes us fat

- Eating fats, allows subsequent fat burning and allows us to lose fat

- Diets of refined and super-refined carbohydrates are killing us and making us ill. We have become carbohydrate lemmings diving off the cliff of metabolic misery

- Fat fuel inhibition reflects the inability to use the fat fueling system

- Fat fuel inhibition reflects our body's addiction to carbohydrates

- Fat fuel inhibition can be reversed

- Fat adaptation is the secret to loosing fat

- Fat adaptation has two phases; food with very low carbohydrates and fasting

- Fat adaptation, while simple to follow, is not easy

- The time required for fat adaptation depends on your diet, fitness and lifestyle

- In the early stages of fat adaptation, you may find irritability, mood swings, brain fog and flu-like symptoms. These settle completely once you are fully fat adapted

CHAPTER 20

THE DIET-WHISPERER SECRETS

"Putting you in personal control of a lean body, smart knowledge and wellness."

Whisperer HQ.

INTRODUCTION

There are three different whisperer plans, that will form part of your armamentarium, depending on your personal circumstances. These are mapped out in detail in the next chapter. You will start with the weight loss phase, the *whisperer-loss* plan. This normally lasts for 12 weeks. It is reasonable to set a target of 1-2 pounds (0.5-1.0 kg) of weight loss per week. Once you reach your target weight you can then adopt the *whisperer-stable* plan to keep you at your desired weight. The *whisperer-active-stable* plan is the same, but with higher protein to meet the demands of those who are more active. And in the long-term, should you err, and put on a few pounds, you can adopt the *whisperer-recover* plan. Our three plans are;

- The diet-whisperer plan for fat loss; *whisperer-loss*

- The diet-whisperer plan to keep you at your target weight; *whisperer-stable*

- The diet-whisperer plan for times in the future when your weight increases; *whisperer-recover*

(figures 20.1, 20.2 and 20.3)

If you have more that 24 pounds (12 kg) to lose, firstly complete the first 0-12-week plan. Then use *whisperer-stable* for 4 weeks and go back and repeat weeks 9-12. Continue this 8-week cycle until you achieve your goals.

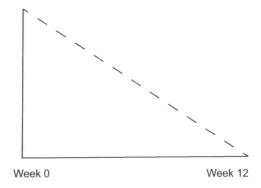

WHISPERER-LOSS PLAN

Week 0   Week 12

Figure 20.1. The whisperer-loss plan.

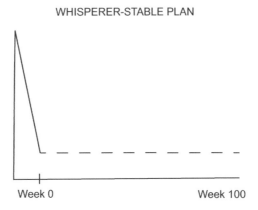

WHISPERER-STABLE PLAN

Week 0   Week 100

Figure 20.2. The whisperer-stable plan.

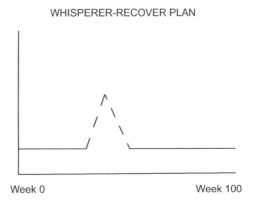

WHISPERER-RECOVER PLAN

Week 0   Week 100

Figure 20.3. The whisperer-recover plan.

And here lie the secrets of the whisperer plans. You will be in control by the time you complete your first 12-week cycle. You will have the knowledge to switch and decide for yourself, how and when you lose your weight. You will be in charge. You will be able to not only help yourself, but others too. You will be a diet-whisperer.

FIVE KEY ELEMENTS

There are five key elements to the whisperer plan and twelve general rules, A-L. The five key elements are;

1. Fat adaptation is used to reverse Fat Fuel Inhibition, also known as carb addiction.

2. Snacking is stopped in all forms.

3. EatSpan is reduced and FastSpan is increased.

4. Refined and super-refined carbohydrates are removed from the diet.

5. You should also follow the advice in the wellness chapter to reduce your cortisol.

Let's look at each of these in more detail

Fat Adaptation

Fat adaption is central to ridding ourselves of excess fat. For the past 100 years, we have fed on excess refined and super-refined carbohydrates, with additional high frequency snacking. We have now learned that our fat burning is switched off by refined carbohydrates and snacking, giving us Fat Fuel Inhibition; another name for carbohydrate addiction. When this goes on for years, we become reliant on glucose as our fuel, and our body is less able to burn fat. Because of this, when our carbohydrate stores run down, we start to feel trembly and weak. At that very moment, when we might have switched our engine from carb-burning to fat-burning, we prevent this by having a cup of tea, or a biscuit. Or a slice of toast, or cake. We do this all day, every day. These habits keep us carbohydrate addicted. In the UK, hospital staff have a constant supply of biscuits bought by grateful patients, a constant supply of toast in rest rooms and a massive problem with staff obesity. I guarantee when you next smell toast in an institution, the staff will be overweight or obese.

Bad teachings and culture have made our hormones confused, leaving us simply unable to burn fat; it is now time to go cold turkey on the carbs and get our hormones, weight and health back.

Two phases of fat adaptation

In the last chapter, I said how tough I found the first few weeks. Well, don't give up, because once fat adaptation is mastered, you will find the new you. Do ask your loved ones to support you as you may become irritable and irrational. Some people get flu like symptoms, stomach upsets and others brain fog. It will be worth it. It is so worthwhile going through the initial suffering.

The time period involved is highly individual, but the first phase will take between 1 and 4 weeks. It really does vary that widely. It is very dependent on your current lifestyle, dietary habits and current fitness. This is why it's harder alone and much easier with the support network of a group of family or friends. Please tell us your experiences online, which will help new members of the whisperer family.

Fat adaptation Phase 1;

- Start by adopting a ketogenic diet, with a maximum of 25-50 grams of carbs each day

- Your diet will have macronutrients in the ratio; carbs <5%; fat 65%; proteins 35%;

- You can calculate exact quantities of dietary macronutrients in grams on the website

- Eat three meals per day and never snack in between

- Be prepared for the symptoms of "keto flu" as your body initially struggles without the refined carbohydrate "hits"; you are effectively going cold turkey on your refined carbs

- Stick with it because only when you have detoxed your carbs will your hormones be back in regular working order. In an emergency, eat an apple, but better still try to ride the storm

- Talk to your family and tell them what you are doing because at times you will be irritable and difficult

- Don't weaken and have that carb hit. You need real strength in the first few weeks and the fewer times you feed your carb addiction with the "rescue apple", the sooner you will be over it

- If you do have to have some fruit, reboot and go again; be kind to yourself

- You can use any of the thousands of keto diets on the internet

- Never snack between meals; the exception is the "rescue apple"

- Do not snack after your last meal in the evening. It is important to fast until breakfast the following day

Fat Adaptation Phase 2;

- You will see in week 4 of the *whisperer-loss* plan, we start to increase the FastSpan and reduce the EatSpan

- To increase you FastSpan, and reduce your EatSpan, you will skip breakfast for one day per week

- The skipping of breakfast will increase in number, week by week, until we omit breakfast completely

- You will gradually move from three meals per day to two meals per day. You are a winner

- We will get you to eat lunch later and your evening meal earlier

- Eating your evening meal just one hour earlier increases your overnight FastSpan significantly

- This all helps with your fat adaptation

- Eventually you will combine breakfast with lunch. Why not just eat the bacon and eggs for lunch instead of having them at breakfast?

- Well done you. After week 8 you will be almost completely fat adapted. Note that fat adaptation continues for many months even up to one year, getting stronger and stronger. The good news is, after the first 8 weeks you are mostly there

- Your fat storage hormones and enzymes will be returning to their healthy state.

No Snacking

It is critical, absolutely critical, that you do not ever snack between meals. Not even a peanut. It is equally critical that nothing is taken between your last meal and getting up in the morning. Apart from water, or black coffee or black tea. As you will learn in the whisperer loss plan, in the first few weeks, you may take a whole fruit, like an apple, if you get really bad carb withdrawal symptoms. The less you do this, the sooner you pull through. You may want to consider decaffeinated tea and coffee, if you are taking drinks around bedtime. Your sleep may well be disturbed in the first week or so, and you may become slightly agitated and moody. Eventually your sleep will not only be better, but thoroughly nourishing, restoring and healing to both mind and body. This is all part of the healing process. You may also find that your bowel habit changes. Keep a check on your thirst and the colour of your urine; if it is darker than a pale straw colour, you may be dehydrated and need more fluids.

EatSpan and FastSpan

You should begin with three low-carb meals per day. You'll feel hungry in waves, and each day this will get better. We find that a few black coffees help in this process, or even water. Personally, at my office desk right now, I have a 2-pint (1 liter) bottle of carbonated water. That and a black coffee will take me through till lunch time, when I shall have a high-fat meal today. Because my hormones are back in balance, I do not get hungry and if I do not feel like lunch, I'll simply omit it. That is how you will be when you are back in total control. For a few weeks, you may find your decision making, or co-ordination sub-optimal. You need to manage the timing and risks of this depending on your career or hobbies!

On the web site, you will see information and graphics about EatSpan and FastSpan, which are interesting to play with. Imagine, you simply eat three meals a day, without snacking, and take your first meal half an hour later, and your last meal half an hour earlier, you will lose 0.5-1.0 pound every week. As a general rule, you try to lengthen your FastSpan and shorten your EatSpan; this has powerful metabolic effects on your hormones and fat burn. FastSpan is the time from the last meal at night, until breakfast. EatSpan is the time from the first meal of the day until the end of the last meal of the day. Any snacks count as meals of course. So, if breakfast is at 07.00, lunch at 12.30, and supper is at 20.00, then you have a FastSpan of 11 hours, and an EatSpan of 13 hours.

The reason for skipping a meal is to shorten the EatSpan and lengthen the FastSpan. Accordingly, the meal skipped should be the first or last meal of the day, as skipping lunch does not achieve this.

Removal of Refined and Super-Refined Carbohydrates from Your Diet

You must keep your daily carbohydrates down to less than 50 grams. Even better is if you can get them below 25 grams. This is fairly standard advice for ketogenic, or "keto" diets and this information is available everywhere. You should by this stage have learned to know what constitutes healthy natural whole food carbs, high in fibre. What grandma refers to as your "greens". These natural carbohydrates are completely acceptable part of any keto, or indeed, whisperer-plan.

What are not acceptable, and therefore have to go, are refined and super-refined carbs. This includes both food and drinks. By eating lots of dietary fibre, you will be feeding your microbiome and keeping your gut healthy; both beneficial for your physical and mental health. Your gut is much more than just a digestive organ, as we saw in the microbiome chapter.

Cortisol

In the wellness chapter, we make many suggestions for lowering your cortisol, which is an important part of your overall weight loss and wellbeing. Looking after your cortisol brings many additional benefits for your mental and physical health too.

TWELVE GENERAL RULES

A. Groups

I'm not going to pretend the first four weeks are going to be easy, but every day, is that one day closer to feeling better. Adopt the plan it with your partner, or even better with a group of friends or family. It really is so much easier to share your experience and give and receive encouragement. Remember at all times, this will change your life for the better. And keep repeating it to yourself.

B. Record Your Food Data

Record your carbs each day. Compare with your group, if you have one, and encourage others as well as yourself. If you fail to meet your goals on day 1, or 4, or 24, put it behind you and get back to concentrating on the day at hand. Look back at your data and count up your success days and stay positive. As coach Wooden says, "make this day your masterpiece". The whisperer encourages you to record the number of meals, EatSpan and FastSpan, and total these each week. There are website tools to help at diet-whisperer.com.

C. Exercise

If you are a keen gym goer, in the initial stages your body will find it difficult to adapt to fat metabolism for fuel. Expect your heart rate to be higher and your peak performance fall compared with your old self. This will improve with time. If you don't normally take regular cardio, consider starting with 15-30-minute walks. If you take these before your first meal of the day, it will help with fat adaptation. A pair of high-quality walking shoes and walking socks is an investment worth its weight in gold, at any point in your life.

If resistance training is your thing, then please continue. But the protein supplements have to go for now. You'll be amazed that you won't have the catastrophic lean tissue loss you feared! If you really, really, really can't bear to be without them, then they must be taken around mealtimes, and reintroduce them after week four. Outside mealtimes they will create havoc with your leptin and insulin recovery and stimulate the normal blood insulin response. Taking them before a meal is also a powerful appetite suppressant.

If you are not into this type of weight training and you're over 35, you should be, as it will help to combat weakness from your sarcopenia. There is no age when you are too old to start weight training. If you can't do press-ups, squats or planks, look them up online and start today. Make them part of your daily routine. Even if you need a chair for your squats, or can only do press-ups from your knees, start today. Small numbers, then build over the 12 weeks.

D. Recording Your Measurements

Measurements and recording them can be very motivational. Spoil yourself and buy a really nice set of bathroom scales and weigh-in on awakening, just once per day and record it. You should buy yourself a tailor's measuring tape. The way to use this is to find the narrowest part of your abdomen, usually just above your belly button, and pull the tape as tight as possible and record that measurement. This gives the very best measurement and reproducibility, by reducing bias from varying levels of tightness. Note this is different from the gentle tightness used for assessing visceral fat from abdominal girth. In this case we are using the measurement to record and compare with consistency. Both your weight and abdominal girth will go up and down. Be patient, because impressive things will happen with time.

E. Using the Whisperer Plans

If you can join friends or make a local diet-whisperer group on social media, this will be a great help. You should bring your partner along as it is very difficult to try and do any diet alone. You will have bad days, bad moods and hunger, but I promise they will pass as your hormones straighten out.

Ask your partner to understand that your metabolic hormonal changes will change your moods initially, sometimes quite severely. There is plenty of guidance on the internet to support your conversion to a ketogenic or paleo diet. Names don't matter; if the carbs are low enough and the fats are high, that's all that matters to make this work. The more your hormones are out of line, the more difficult the first week will be. If you have had a really bad diet for a long time and are carb addicted, you will have a degree of "cold turkey" from your refined carb withdrawal. You may even need to take a week away from work.

F. Dirty Versus Clean Keto

There are two versions of high fats that can be used together or on their own depending on your current diet. If you are already eating well, we recommend you continue with "clean" keto. That is your fats come from the healthiest sources like oily-fish, avocados, eggs, nuts and olives. You will be cooking with and using nut oils and the best extra virgin olive oils. This is the basis of the Mediterranean diet and there are many pluses to including this as part of the whisperer plan. Just as long as you keep the carbs low enough and aim for below 25 grams.

If your normal diet is rich in meat, we recommend you continue at least for the first 12 weeks, with "dirty" keto as explained below. Over the months, convert yourself from dirty to clean, one foodstuff at a time, but never suddenly, as you will give up quickly. If you eat bacon, sausage, mushroom, tomato and eggs for breakfast, carry on. Just no bread and make sure those carbs stay below 25 grams. Cook in healthy oils, like nut oil, even lard or butter, rather than seed-based vegetable oil filled with omega-6s. There can be problems with olive oils on very high heat, so I do my fry ups with butter and olive oil over a gentle flame. If you can't or don't want to convert to clean keto foods, don't worry as the plan still works and you can think about that much later.

If dirty keto is your norm, we recommend you slowly convert after the first

12 weeks to partially clean (salmon, oily fish, unrefined vegetables), but it is important to try and enjoy your food, for long term success. If you prefer to stay on "dirty keto" then please continue unabated. There is plenty of time for the nuances ahead; let's get this bit right first. It is much, much healthier than a high carbohydrate diet and will allow you to reduce weight and get healthier. We just know that clean keto is that bit better still. That's a choice for you and it's great you have got this far. And either route, you end up with your hormones straightened out and your body able to burn fat.

Remember to drink two to three litres of water per day. Black tea and black coffee can be a welcome substitute as you will find out. Sparkling water also makes a change.

G. Foods banned completely for the first 8 weeks;

- All flour based or coated foods

- All pasta-based foods

- Beer, sweet wines and prosecco (see general rule "J" below)

- Bread of all types

- Breakfast cereals

- Cordials

- Diet foods

- Fruit; apart from rescue apples, no fruit for the first eight weeks

- Fruit juices of any kind

- High Fructose Corn Syrup containing foods; look for HFCS on labels

- Legumes (beans) these may be reintroduced later

- Noodles

- Pizzas

- Potato based foods, including chips, fries and crisps (potato skins are allowed)

- Puddings and ice cream

- Pulses (chickpeas and lentils) these may be reintroduced later

- Rice of all kinds

- Soda drinks including energy drinks and diet sodas

- Sugar including pseudonyms and substitutes like honey, molasses, dates, raisins

- Sugar, sweets, candy, chocolate bars, energy bars

- Sweeteners, both natural and artificial

- Vegetable oils high in omega-6s

H. Whisperer Allowed Foods for first 8 weeks of *whisperer-loss*.

Total carbohydrates must be less than 25-50 grams per day;

- Avocado

- Bacon, burger patties (no bread)

- Beansprouts

- Berries in small amounts (blueberries, blackberries, raspberries, strawberries)

- Black tea and coffee without sweeteners

- Bone broths

- Broccoli, kale, spinach and cauliflower

- Butter and Ghee

- Cheese

- Coconut oil

- Cod liver oil 2 teaspoons daily or Chlorella or spirulina

- Cooked and preserved meats (hams, sausages, salami etc.)

- Cream; full fat only

- Eggs

- Fish and shellfish

- Meat and poultry

- Milk full fat only

- Multivitamin tablets

- Natural Greek style yogurt

- Nuts, in modest servings

- Olive oil (extra virgin best), canola (rapeseed) oil, nut oil

- Olives

- Onions, garlic, herbs, spices and chilies

- Potato skins

- Red and green bell peppers, green beans, celery

- Salads

- Seeds such as flax, sesame, pumpkin and chia

- Shirataki noodles

- Soups; low in carbs

- Sweet potatoes

- Vinegar all types

- Vitamin D

- Water

- Zucchini and Cucumber

I. Whisperer General Principles

- Consume high quality, whole foods

- Abandon refined and super-refined carbohydrates

- Maintain adequate fluid intake at all times

- Really work hard to increase your PUFA omega-3s

- Limit your PUFA omega-6s to 17 grams per day for men and 12 grams for women

- Supplements are fine, when our whole foods are not nutrient rich enough to supply us, particularly multivitamins, vitamin D and fish oils

- Avoid low-fat foods, because of added carbs. They are both fattening and unhealthy, particularly if they contain HFCS

- Full fat foods and fats in general do not increase weight

- Removing fats from the diet is a bad thing and is associated with weight gain and Fat Fuel Inhibition

- Snacking is called a meal and prevents fat burn

- Snacking is a sign of poor metabolic health. Working to stop snacking habits, leads to positive changes in metabolic and fat storage hormones

- Fat adaptation, allows us to feel better and get the benefits from fasting

- Your body should be fully fat adapted before progressing to intermittent fasting

- Reducing the EatSpan and lengthening the FastSpan leads to significant weight loss

- Fasting is associated with autophagy, wellness and reduced aging

J. Alcohol

Note for people who really cannot give up their alcohol, beverages from best to worst are as follows. And if you normally socialize in drinking "rounds" replace your beer with a single shot as this will reduce your drinking significantly. Do whatever you can in the first four weeks to drink as little as possible. Drinking will return. Remember, your tolerance to alcohol will be much lower and whenever you have alcohol on board, the body will deal with this toxin, rather than fat burn. The following are keto and fat adaptation friendly;

1. Vodka with carbonated "sparkling" water and lime with a shot of bitters.

2. Gin (or Vodka) and Tonic. Watch the carb count.

3. Red wine.

4. Champagne.

K. Important Considerations

There is light at the end of the tunnel. In week 9, we will show you how to keep your hormones in order, whilst affording yourself some treat meals. A pizza, a curry or your favourite Thai. We will show you how these can be an enjoyable part of a healthy eating plan. We will show you how to incorporate these into your plan, when you have reached your target weight.

L. Intermittent Fasting Days and Treat Meals

- For simplicity, we have been quite didactic in the plans. We do understand that in real life you have to be flexible, to meet the demands of work and family life. So, we suggest you sit down on a Sunday and plan the week ahead choosing your own days for fasting and treat meals.

- Each week the plan will have two key factors for you to follow, whilst observing the guiding principles above.

- Your food, which will tell you where you are on the plan for fats, proteins and carbs.

- Your EatSpan and FastSpan, and how to change these for optimum fat loss.

CHAPTER 21

THE DIET-WHISPERER PLANS

"To err is human, to forgive divine"

Alexander Pope, 1711.

INTRODUCTION

In the previous chapters, you have gained all the knowledge required to apply the *whisperer-loss* plan to yourself, family and friends. You have learned the ground rules. On Sunday every week, sit down and plan your week ahead. You are now on your road to taking back control of your weight and physical and mental health. The road to a new you.

The first 8 weeks change weekly but are quite didactic and simple to follow. The plans are laid out in table form so you can easily follow them. On week 9, you start to have choices over which days you have treats and which days you increase you FastSpan. Ultimately, the only way you can keep control of your weight, is to understand your food, and how it affects your metabolic hormones. You will be able to choose your weight, get there and stay there. At that stage you will be in total control and able to continue at your chosen weight forever, using the *whisperer-stable* plan. To err is common, and we all do, but the whisperer plans are forgiving, allowing you simply get back to target using *whisperer-recover.*

There are many helpful tools to track your progress on our website; diet-whisperer.com.

WHISPERER-LOSS

Terminology

- Macros; means the percentage of each macronutrient in your meals C5 means 5% carbohydrates, F65 means 65% fats and P35 means 35% proteins

- To convert these to grams, you can use the website at diet-whisperer.com

- If you wish to perform the conversion manually, use the formula % number/100, so P35 becomes 35/100 or 0.35, then multiple your BMI (daily calories) by this figure. To get to grams simply divide the resulting number by 4 for carbs and proteins and 9 for fats. There you have your grams for each macronutrient

For the next 12 weeks, you should be recording the total number of meals per week, remembering that any snack including your rescue apple is a meal, and your weekly total FastSpan and EatSpan.

Treat meals are anything you choose to eat, maybe a pizza or in my case Pakistani or Bangladeshi food. We avoid all super-refined carbs, but refined carbs are allowed as part of our treat meals. So, pizza bases, chapatis, burger buns, other breads, rice and pasta are all allowed as part of our treat meals, beginning week 9.

WEEK 1

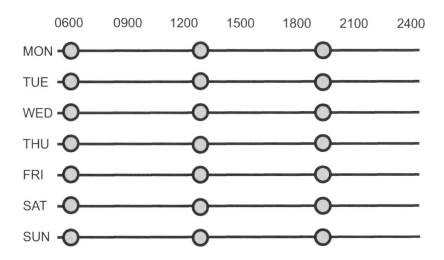

Figure 21.1. EatSpan for Whisperer-loss week 1
Total meals per week = 21

Food;

- Carbs: fat: protein in the ratio C5:F65:P35. Keeping carbs below 25-50 grams
- No refined or super-refined carbs
- No snacking before or after meals, or between last meal and breakfast
- 3 litres of fluid per day in the form of unsweetened black coffee, tea or water
- In the first few weeks if you find carbohydrate withdrawal tough, an occasional whole fruit may be eaten, such as an apple. We call this your "rescue apple". Give yourself 5 whole fruits for emergencies in the first week
- Stop drinking alcohol (see previous chapter)
- Total meal number = 21

EatSpan and FastSpan

- 3 meals per day taken at anytime

WEEK 2

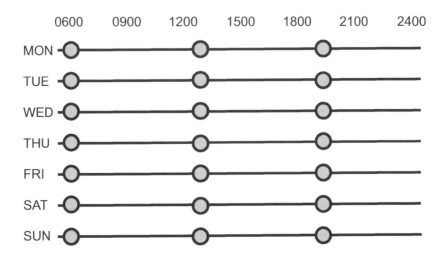

Figure 21.2. EatSpan for Whisperer-loss week 2
Total meals per week = 21

Food

- Unchanged

- 3 rescue apples permitted for the week

- Total meal number = 21

EatSpan and FastSpan

- 3 meals per day taken at any time

WEEK 3

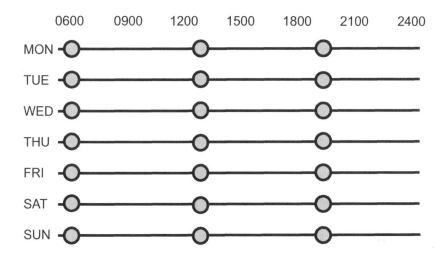

Figure 21.3. EatSpan for Whisperer-loss week 3
Total meals per week = 21

Food

- Unchanged

- 1 rescue apple permitted for the week

- Total meal number = 21

EatSpan and FastSpan

- 3 meals per day taken at any time

WEEK 4

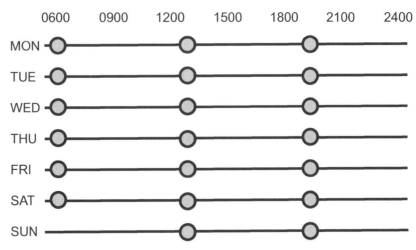

Figure 21.4. EatSpan for Whisperer-loss week 4.
Total meals per week = 20

Food

- Unchanged

- 0 rescue apples this week!

- Total meal number = 20

EatSpan and FastSpan

- This week you will miss breakfast on Sunday

- 3 meals per day taken at any time

You are now at the end of your first 4-week block and will have lost 4-10 pounds (2-5 kg). Very well done; you're on the way to real success. It will get progressively easier, although you may still have the odd rough day. Your hormones will be really getting back to their happy normal state by now. Well done from all at whisperer HQ.

WEEK 5

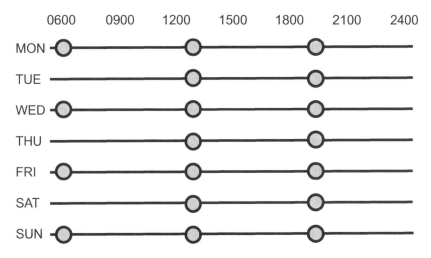

Fig. 21.5 EatSpan for Whisperer-loss week 5. Meals = 18

You're now feeling more comfortable, fat adapting well and seeing significant weight loss. Now you are into the next phase and we will start to change the meal timings.

Food

- Carbs: fat: protein unchanged at C5:F65:P35. Keep those carbs under 25-50 grams
- 3 litres of fluid per day in the form of black coffee, tea or water
- No snacking with refined carbs
- Refrain from drinking alcohol
- Total meal number = 18

EatSpan and FastSpan

- 3 meals per day most days, but you will skip breakfast on 3 mornings
- On the two meal days see how you have increased the previous night's FastSpan
- Also your EatSpan is down and your hormones can now burn through fat

You are now seeing some days with three magical ingredients. Your EatSpan is down, your FastSpan is up, and some days you've reduced your number of meals from 3 to 2. Now you are making tangible progress. Well done.

WEEK 6

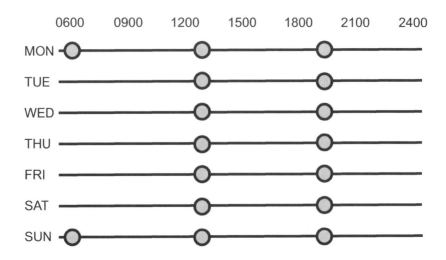

Figure 21.6. EatSpan for Whisperer-loss week 6.
Total meals per week = 16

Keep the faith, as there are some treats in 3 weeks' time.

Food

- Unchanged

- Total meal number = 16

EatSpan and FastSpan

- 3 meals per day for 2 days; and on 5 days skip breakfast

- Thereby increasing your weekly FastSpan

- Thereby decreasing your weekly EatSpan

- Thereby reducing your weekly total number of meals

You are making great progress. Well done.

WEEK 7

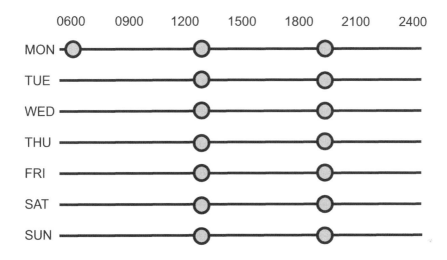

Figure 21.7. EatSpan for Whisperer-loss week 7.
Total meals per week = 15

Keep the faith, as there are some treats in 2 weeks' time.

Food

- Unchanged

- Total meal number = 15

EatSpan and FastSpan

- 3 meals per day for 1 day; and on 6 days skip breakfast

Don't forget to keep your daily EatSpan and FastSpan hours and tot them up at the end of the week. You are making real progress. Well done.

WEEK 8

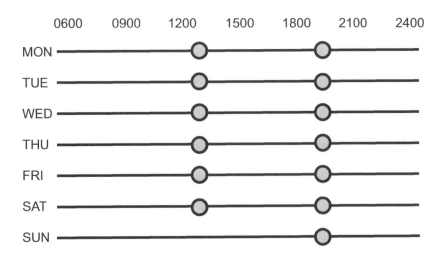

Figure 21.8. EatSpan for Whisperer-loss week 8.
Total meals per week = 13

Keep the faith, as there are some welcome treats next week.

Food

- Unchanged

- Total meal number = 13

EatSpan and FastSpan

- Two meals every day on all except one day when you will not only skip breakfast, but lunch too

- That means you will do your first 24-hour fast. This is a big and significant day; well done

- Try your best to reduce you EatSpan as well. Even 30-60 minutes will make a difference, as your weekly totals will show; that is brunch later or evening meal earlier

You are now at the end of your second 4-week block. Well done. You will have lost between 8 and 16 pounds (4-8 kg). You are now getting your hormones realigned and feeling better about the whole situation. I hope you take real encouragement from your success. And have a look at how your figures have improved; EatSpan and total meals per week are down, and FastSpan is up.

WEEK 9

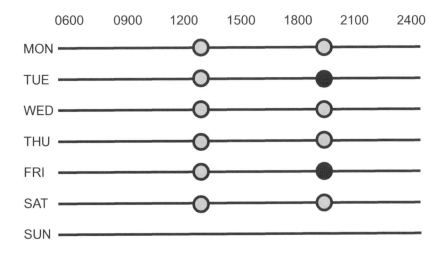

Figure 21.9. EatSpan for Whisperer-loss week 9.
Total meals per week = 12. Note treat meals x2

Welcome to week 9, the start of your last 4-week *whisperer-loss* block. This is where you put your new hormonal balance to the test and see how capable your body is of managing with longer periods without food. Thankfully, we will reintroduce two treat meals this week too. Lunch or supper, and whatever is your favourite food. You may also have an alcoholic drink with your meal. Beware this requires careful planning. It is great to fast for a long period after your treat meal. But, if a lot of alcohol is consumed, this can lead to low blood sugar the next day. Under these circumstances, plan a luxury brunch the following day, followed by your fast, until lunch time the next day, or if you can, until supper. Some people find this stage quite nerve-wracking, but rest assured it is perfectly safe for heathy individuals to fast. Science has shown fasts of three weeks not only to be safe, but positively beneficial. We are not suggesting this for you, but just be reassured, fasting is as old as the hills; we've just forgotten the benefits. When you get the hang of this, it will change your life forever. You will be in charge of your body and health for ever more, in just 4-weeks' time. Choose your day this week for the long fast. I usually go from Saturday night until Monday evening meal. Some weeks I go from Sunday brunch until Tuesday or even Wednesday evening meal. It's a very powerful tool to learn as you will discover.

Food

- Carbs/ fat/ protein 5%/ 65%/ 35% for all but two treat meals
- 3 litres of fluid per day in the form of black coffee, tea or water
- Two treat lunches or evening meals, with alcohol should you so desire
- Really enjoy your treat meals
- Total meal number = 12

EatSpan and FastSpan

- Two meals each day, leading up to the 42-hour fast
- One fast is for 42 hours, from Saturday evening meal until Monday lunchtime.

It is one of the greatest moments when you realise you can fast without hunger or symptoms. You know you are on the way. Every fast gets easier and easier, as you get stronger and healthier. Think of all the anti-inflammatory changes in your body and brain. All that anti-aging and autophagy. All that renewal and regeneration.

WEEK 10

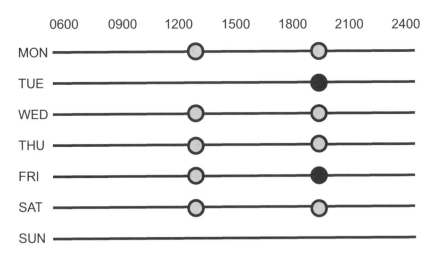

Fig. 21.10 Meals = 11. Treat meals = 2

Your first 42-hour plus fast was last week. It will be no big deal by now. So, choose again this week, but two days. On other days you should be eating only two meals each day, at lunch and evening, with breakfast now completely omitted from your diet. On this week, if you don't need lunch one day, don't take it. Only foolish rules state we eat when not requiring to. So, try to miss a lunch this week too. You will be noticing by now that your shape is changing considerably.

Food

- Carbs/ fat/ protein 5%/ 65%/ 35% for all but two treat meals
- 3 litres of fluid per day in the form of black coffee, tea or water
- Stop drinking alcohol, except at the two treat meals
- Total meal number = 11

EatSpan and FastSpan

- 2 meals per day, on 5 days
- One fast for 24 hours from Monday evening to your treat meal on Tuesday evening
- At the end of this week is another 42-hour fast

WEEK 11

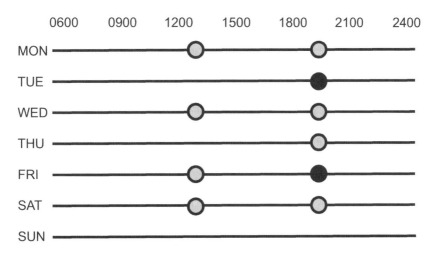

Fig. 21.11 Meals = 10. Treat meals = 2

On 4 days you will be eating only two meals each day, at lunch and evening, with breakfast now completely omitted from your diet. This week you will miss 3 lunches too. You will be noticing by now that your shape is changing considerably. As a general rule applicable to the rest of your life, when you come to any mealtime and don't feel hungry, don't eat. Only foolish rules state we eat when we don't need or want to.

Food

- Carbs/ fat/ protein 5%/ 65%/ 35% for all but two treat meals
- 3 litres of fluid per day in the form of black coffee, tea or water
- Stop drinking alcohol, except at the two treat meals
- Total meal number = 10

EatSpan and FastSpan

- 2 meals a day for 4 days
- Two 24-hour fasts during the week
- One 48-hour fast at the end of this week

WEEK 12

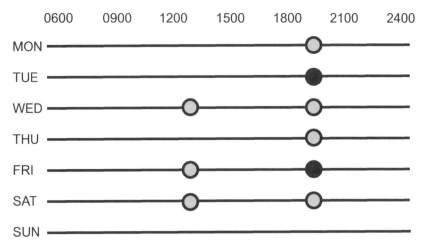

Fig. 21.12 Meals = 9. Treat meals = 2

On 3 days this week you will be eating only two meals each day. You will miss 4 lunches too.

Food

- Carbs/ fat/ protein 5%/ 65%/ 35% for all but two treat meals
- 3 litres of fluid per day in the form of black coffee, tea or water
- Stop drinking alcohol, except at the two treat meals
- Total meal number = 9

EatSpan and FastSpan

- 2 meals per day for 3 days
- Two 24-hour fasts
- At the end of this week you will also have a 42-hour to 48-hour fast

This is really where we hand over and you take the controls. Where you utilize all the skills you've learned to create your own path going forwards, enjoying your fasting days as much as your food days. This balance will stay with you for life, completely changing your relationship with food and gaining a fantastic hormonal balance, as well as a sense of physical and mental wellbeing. You have completed your whisperer plan and have regained your feelings of wellness. Well done and congratulations. Welcome to the family new whisperer.

WHISPERER-LOSS PLAN

	Week 1	Week 2	Week 3	Week 4
Macro C5:F65;P35	Yes	Yes	Yes	Yes
Refined carbs	No	No	No	No
Super-refined carbs	No	No	No	No
Snacks	No	No	No	No
Daily 4-6 pints (2-3l) fluids	Yes	Yes	Yes	Yes
Rescue apple	5	3	1	0
Alcohol	No	No	No	No
Breakfasts	7	7	7	6
Lunches	7	7	7	7
Evening meals	7	7	7	7
Meals per week	21	21	21	20
Treat meals per week	0	0	0	0

Figure 21.13. Weeks 1-4 of the whisperer-loss plan.

WHISPERER-LOSS PLAN

	Week 5	Week 6	Week 7	Week 8
Macro C5:F65;P35	Yes	Yes	Yes	Yes
Refined carbs	No	No	No	No
Super-refined carbs	No	No	No	No
Snacks	No	No	No	No
Daily 4-6 pints (2-3l) fluids	Yes	Yes	Yes	Yes
Rescue apple	No	No	No	No
Alcohol	No	No	No	No
Breakfasts	4	2	1	0
Lunches	7	7	7	6
Evening meals	7	7	7	7
Meals per week	18	16	15	13
Treat meals per week	0	0	0	0

Figure 21.14. Weeks 5-8 of the whisperer-loss plan.

WHISPERER-LOSS PLAN

	Week 9	Week 10	Week 11	Week 12
Macro C5:F65;P35	Yes	Yes	Yes	Yes
Refined carbs	Treats	Treats	Treats	Treats
Super-refined carbs	No	No	No	No
Snacks	No	No	No	No
Daily 4-6 pints (2-3l) fluids	Yes	Yes	Yes	Yes
Rescue apple	No	No	No	No
Alcohol	Treats	Treats	Treats	Treats
Breakfasts	0	0	0	0
Lunches	6	5	4	3
Evening meals	6	6	6	6
Meals per week	12	11	10	9
Treat meals per week	2	2	2	2

Figure 21.15. Weeks 9-12 of the whisperer-loss plan. In these four weeks, longer 48 hour periods of fasting are achieved. Note that some refined carbohydrates and alcohol are allowed with treat meals.

WHISPERER STABLE AND WHISPERER-ACTIVE-STABLE

Long term weight stability and metabolic health are dependent on keeping your food and hormones aligned, and in harmony with your body. To do this is very simple and easily understood. It is a combination of EatSpan, FastSpan and food type. You now have all the skills to combine these and get your perfect balance. Your treat meals will go up and down each week depending on work, play or holidays with the family.

The macronutrient composition of the *whisperer-stable* plan is C40;F40;P20. The protein here represents 1g/kg per day. We avoid refined carbs except for treat meals. We have no limit on unrefined vegetables. If you are exercising and or doing resistance training, we recommend increasing your protein up to 2g/kg per day. This equates to approximately 40% protein. This would change your ratios to whisperer-active-stable,C30;F30;P40. This can be calculated on the website.

An important part of both *whisperer-stable* and *whisperer-active-stable* is that we follow a rule of thumb for those delicious carbs that mess up our hormones. Refined carbohydrates are allowed at treat meals, three times per week. Super-refined carbohydrates are super unhealthy, so we reserve those for occasional treats, by which we mean on your Birthday! That is, once each year.

I could never live a life without my treat meals out with friends, drinking beer and wine. I'm never going to be that fully compliant person. My weeks are too up and down, and I'm too spontaneous to have to worry all the time about what I eat and drink. My baseline tendency is to do the wrong thing with food and drink. The wrong things, at the wrong times and too frequently for comfort. But I'm happy with that, as I have found my happy medium, whereby I can fast for two to three days per week and enjoy it very much. But also enjoy my treat foods and drink. This allows my weight to stay stable.

Whisperer-stable and *whisperer-active-stable* are very much about you. About you finding your personal balance. If you're in a relationship, you might do what Monique and I do; sit down and make a plan that works well for us both. Monique and I eat together 70% of the time. The other 30% we do our own thing. My *whisperer-stable* is two lunches per week, when I pick up some treats from a local bakery at lunchtime. I sit in my car, parked in the countryside, reading the paper and listening to the radio. I know, its not perfect, but it's my way of finding a balance that works for me. My weight has been stable for twelve months now and I absolutely love that I can combine treats, like curries, naan breads and sandwiches, with sensible keto and paleo foods and long intermittent fasts. I cannot even begin to tell you on a Sunday morning how much I enjoy my fast until Tuesday or Wednesday evening, every single week. Those deep, nourishing and satisfying sleeps. I love to do my long meditations on those days. This week on Monday, I lost some computer data, that took me all day to recover. On Monday night I was quite agitated after a very frustrating day. So, Monique made a decision to compulsorily open Bar Chell, where we sit in our open plan kitchen, on bar stools boozing, laughing and chatting. We ate leftover meats from the fridge, with mainly pickles, predominantly green chili pickle. It was lovely and just what the doctor(s) ordered. We awoke on Tuesday with whacking hangovers, following an unhealthy number of gin and tonics. And according to the detritus the next day, quite a few bottles of beers too and about a kilo of shrapnel in the form of pistachio nut shells.

So, I hope you now get this whole plan. It's for normal humans that err. It is for you, me and Monique. Each week we are dodging bullets, but not trying to rid ourselves of all of them. There may be the occasional wound or casualty, but we continue to be stable, enjoying life and keeping as safe as possible. If you prefer to be perfect, then you're a better person than me. And I admire you. If you're after the right balance of treats, and fasts, you now have all the skills to make your own whisperer plan.

People all over the world have successfully tuned their intermittent fasting and feasting days to suit. Let me give you some examples;

- Alternate days fasting

- Fasting daily Monday to Friday with one meal per day

- Fasting daily 7 days a week, with 3 meals a day for holidays

WHISPERER-STABLE PLAN

	Every week	Notes
Macro C40:F40;P20	Yes	
Refined carbs	3	Treat meals only
Super-refined carbs	No	Once in a blue moon
Snacks	No	
Daily 4-6 pints (2-3l) fluids	Yes	
Fasts of 48 hours or longer	1	And one 3-5 day fast
Alcohol	3	Treat meals only
Breakfasts	0	
Lunches	3	
Evening meals	6	
Meals per week	9	
Treat meals per week	3	

Figure 21.13. Weekly whisperer-stable plan. This allows for one fast each week of over 48 hours. Each month, this fast is extended to one longer 3-5 day fast, to reap the regenerative benefits of a longer fast. Alcohol may be taken along with the 3 treat meals.

- Fasting for 36 hours once weekly combined with 1 and 2 meals on alternate days

- Fasting for 48 hours once weekly

- 16;8 which means a FastSpan of 16 hours each day and an EatSpan of 8 hours

- Or Michael Moseley's 5:2 or a 4:3 or alternate both

So, once you achieve your target, you simply balance your low carbs with treats, and you personalize your EatSpan and FastSpan to suit you.

There are an infinite number of variations that can suit each individual. I have a close friend who used the whisperer plan to achieve his target weight and now eats one meal every day, alternating low-carb and treats. If he puts weight on, he fasts for 2-3 days, which is perfectly safe.

You are now officially your own diet-whisperer. Keep whispering and join our chat group through the website. Spread the word and make the world a better place. Keep up those daily measurements and tweak your diet, EatSpan and FastSpan as necessary. But most of all enjoy your new life, with treats without guilt, and your new joie de vivre.

And please, keep the wonderful messages coming on the website, and keep in touch. Let us know your story.

WHISPERER RECOVER

You hardly need me to guide you through this at all by this stage. But if you have a food or alcohol wobble and put on a few pounds, take a breath and regroup. Maybe you were on holiday and ate gorgeous food, with lovely wine and put on a few pounds. No worries at all. Take time and include wellness, meditation if you like, but certainly good sleep in your recovery plan.

Regroup and remember you have at least two weeks before your fat adaptation is lost. So, if your blowout is less than two weeks, go back to your *whisperer-stable* plan, cut down the alcohol, or go for keto suitable

WHISPERER-ACTIVE-STABLE PLAN

	Every week	Notes
Macro C30:F30;P40	Yes	higher protein
Refined carbs	3	Treat meals only
Super-refined carbs	No	Once in a blue moon
Snacks	No	
Daily 4-6 pints (2-3l) fluids	Yes	
Fasts of 48 hours or longer	1	And one 3-5 day fast
Alcohol	3	Treat meals only
Breakfasts	0	
Lunches	3	
Evening meals	6	
Meals per week	9	
Treat meals per week	3	

Figure 21.14. Weekly whisperer-active-stable plan, for people who train, increasing the protein intake. This allows for one fast each week over 48 hours. Each month, this fast is extended to one longer 3-5 day fast, to reap the regenerative benefits of a longer fast. Alcohol may be taken along with the 3 treat meals.

drinking. Then add in a few long fasts and you'll soon be on the road to recovery.

If your blowout was for more than two weeks, then go back to 1-2 weeks of strict fat adaptation. Then ease back into your preferred *whisperer-stable* plan and add in 1-3-day fasts until you get back on track. If you wish you can do a couple of really long fasts of 3-7 days. The important thing is that you know how to do all this, that it is perfectly safe, and it's you that is in charge. Today, tomorrow and forever.

From Monique, me and all at whisperer HQ, welcome. :-)

You are now a diet-whisperer.

CHAPTER 22

WELLNESS

"It is Health that is real Wealth and not Pieces of Gold and Silver"

Mahatma Gandhi

INTRODUCTION

Wellness means that your mind, your body and your relationships are in harmony. Wellness is a positive state, encapsulating all aspects of your life. Achieving wellness in the modern world is not an easy quest. Our modern world draws us constantly away from wellness. We work long hours, there is pressure to perform, and we're under stress. Our family, our friends and our communities all bear the impact of our stresses. Wellness is the opposite of stress. There are many factors that you can control and modify in your life; factors that are proven to improve your wellness.

LIFESPAN, HEALTHSPAN AND DISEASESPAN

Christopher Hitchens, polemicist, writer and intellectual, died at the age of 62. Known for his wit, style and originality, he was a regular figure on the public lecture and debating circuit. A smoker and drinker, he developed terminal throat cancer. He discussed illness and death, in an intimate interview with Jeremy Paxman.

When asked if he feared death, his answer was "Er, there's nothing to be afraid of. I won't know that I'm dead". And that rings true, we really aren't afraid of death; after all, we know that we are all going to die. He continued, "I'm afraid of a sordid death, that I would die in an ugly and squalid way and cancer can be pitiless in that way". And there's the rub, death is inevitable,

WELLNESS

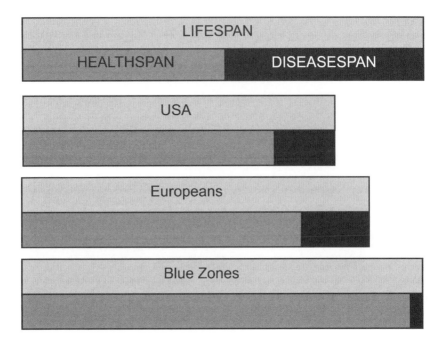

Figure 22.1. Lifespan, healthspan and diseasespan in the US, Europe and the Blue Zones.

but what many of us are afraid of, is the process of dying. We want to die well, and we don't want a bad death. Ideally, we want to stay healthy right up to our death.

This concept is encapsulated in the concept that lifespan is how long you live; from birth to death. Lifespan can be divided into two parts; healthspan and diseasespan. healthspan is the proportion of your life when you are completely well. You do not take tablets and you do not have any disease. You enter diseasespan when you develop a long-term illness such as high blood pressure, metabolic syndrome or even as I sometimes frighteningly hear, a "touch of diabetes".

A long healthspan is ideal, with no diseases, no tablets and no hospital visits. People in the world's Blue Zones have long healthspans, with very short diseasespans. We want our lifespan to be composed of health, not illness. This may well be the reason that you are reading this book. The idea of years of suffering from a raft of inflammatory diseases including dementia, diabetes and cancer, followed by blindness, impotence, incontinence and leg amputations is horrifying. We want to help you keep your diseasespan as short as possible (figure 22.1).

BLUE ZONES

There are a number of places in the world where people live to a very ripe old age. These places are called Blue Zones.[136] In Blue Zones, there are the highest number of people reaching 100 years and older, in the world. And furthermore, they are well; they do not have long-term diseases. They are not living with diseases and frailty. Ikarians, who live on the Greek island of Ikaria, one of the Blue Zones, are almost entirely free of dementia and other long-term diseases.

People in Blue Zones have long lifespans, long healthspans and very short diseasespans. They are not spending the end of their lives grappling with poor health. They live a long healthy life, then they die. The inhabitants of the Blue Zones are amazing examples of people who demonstrate wellness (figure 22.2).

Researchers have tried to analyze the reasons for health and longevity in these places.[136] It is a little more complicated than a simple list of lifestyle features. Could it be genetic? Genes do play a part, but only a small part in determining longevity. Twin studies have shown that longevity is 25% genetic and 75% relates to other causes.[137,138] Environmental influences, such as diet and lifestyle play a big role. Those who live in Blue Zones share certain lifestyle characteristics.

The communities in which they live are very social communities. There is widespread engagement in the community. The right tribe supports healthy behaviors. There is a strong sense of family. There is commitment to a life partner, and they invest time in their children and family members who live nearby. Nicoyan centenarians tend to live with their families, laugh a lot

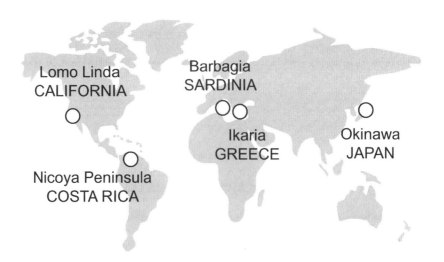

Figure 22.2. The world's Blue Zones.

and spend time with younger people. They frequently visit their neighbors. A strong sense of purpose is a common theme in Blue Zone communities. People feel needed and valued, and they also want to contribute.

Blue Zone diets are rich in vegetables and plant foods; beans, and lentils are the cornerstone of diets. Meat is eaten as a celebration, in small amounts once per week. Other foods consumed regularly include nuts, fish, legumes and whole grains.

Periodic fasting and or calorie restriction is common in Blue Zones. Ikarians are Greek Orthodox Christians. Their religious calendar calls for fasting for almost half the year. Fewer calories may be contributing to people's longevity in the Blue Zones.[139] The Okinawans follow a mealtime rule called "Hara hacki bu". They stop eating when they are 80% full, not 100% full. We know our satiety hormone leptin takes 20 minutes to reach our brain's satiety center. Eating slowly, allows our hormones time to make us feel satisfied and full. The smallest meal is eaten last, in the early afternoon or evening, with nothing thereafter.

Exercise is a way of life; it is part of their day. But no-one is going to the gym. Their environment nudges them to move. The farmers in Sardinia, live on hillsides, raise farm animals and walk long distances to work; moving is part of their lives. People in Blue Zones have gardens, grow their own food and tend their gardens by hand.

And here's a real bonus. People in Blue Zones drink alcohol in moderate amounts. Red wine consumption is particularly common in the Icarian and Sardinian Blue Zones. Moderate consumption is one to two glasses per day. In some studies, though not all, red wine has been linked with health benefits. This is attributed to antioxidants of which resveratrol, a plant antioxidant, is present in some red wines. The Sardinian Cannonau red wine has been shown to have high levels of antioxidants.[140] Unfortunately, you don't get double the benefits if you double your intake; more wine is not better. If you exceed moderate alcohol consumption, this will have the opposite effect.[141]

We can all learn a lot about life looking at the communities in Blue Zones. The world has discovered the secret to wellness. Using the principles learned, Blue Zones projects are under way, to help people live longer and better lives. Fort Worth in Texas, Spencer City in Iowa and Beach Cities in California, have all reaped benefits from implementing these changes. Starting with the environment, the project moves to engagement of the community and transformation of lives.[142] We can all learn a lot by copying from the people who live in the Blue Zones.

SPIRITUALITY, RELAXATION AND MEDITATION (BY PAUL)

I was bought up a Christian, but more latterly, I have got to rather like Buddhism and have studied it in some detail. I like the 'live and let live mantra' of Buddhism. I also like the principles of 'love thy neighbor as thyself' in Christianity. I also very much enjoy meditation. For my meditation I use Headspace, the online guided meditation company founded by Andy Puddicombe, after he returned to Western life from his life as a Buddhist Monk.

Quite often these days I meditate without guidance. I do it as soon as I wake up and have a room in my house with a small Buddhist shrine, with little life mementos on it. I tend to do my stretching and yoga before meditation. Stretching is such a beautiful activity and being more supple makes for a real feeling of youth and well-being. My regime gets as short as 20 minutes for both, and over an hour if I'm feeling very contemplative. Meditating daily has been shown to lengthen our telomeres, those little protective ends to our shoelace like chromosomes. And when our telomeres are gone, we follow soon after.

Every day, I try to become a better person. I often fail, usually mildly, but occasionally miserably. And when I do, I try to remember lessons from people or books that inspire me to improve. When I was in my early 40s, I commissioned two bedside cabinets, each 900 mm, approximately one yard, cubed. They carry all our current books for bedtime reading. There is one book always present and that is The Holy Bible.

I am a great fan of the late John Wooden.[135] He was an uber successful basketball coach and always tried to live his life in a good Christian manner. His father gave him some rules to live by. In his book "John Wooden" he says, "I am a common man who is true to his beliefs." His father Joshua, taught him and his brothers, and subsequently me, to live by his two sets of threes;

1. Never lie.

2. Never cheat.

3. Never steal.

The first set needs no explanation. The second set were about dealing with adversity.

1. Don't whine.

2. Don't complain.

3. Don't make excuses.

When John left school, his dad gave him a two-dollar bill. He said, if you hang onto this, you'll never be broke. On a card he wrote down his mantra for leading a good life.

- Be true to yourself

- Help others

- Make each day your masterpiece

- Drink deeply from good books, especially the bible

- Make friendship a fine art

- Build a shelter against a rainy day

- Pray for guidance and count and give thanks for your blessings every day

When he gave John the note, he said try to live up to these every day. As John says, "I wish I could say I have lived up to them. Over the years I have tried."

A wonderful man.

And that's it. I try to meditate daily, do my yoga and stretching, drink less alcohol, eat more omega-3s and take my vitamin D spray. I fail a lot, and you may well too. But re-boot and try again tomorrow. Try your best to make each day a masterpiece. All you can do is try. And what is truly to me the wonderment of Variable Intermittent Fasting, it allows us, just like coach Wooden, to reboot and start over again today. If last night was curry and beer, then make today your masterpiece.

GOD (BACK TO MONIQUE)

Pascal was a great mathematician, one of the founders of probability theory. His gambit or Pascal's wager was this: "If you bet on God and you were wrong, you have only finite losses (praying, going to church etc.). But if you bet on God and win you stand to win infinite gains". Even Christopher Hitchens, a renowned antitheist, labeled Pascal a huckster for this wager. Of the world's population, 84% identify with a religious group.[143] Religion is on the wane in Europe and North America but is growing virtually everywhere elsewhere in the world.

In all Blue Zones, centenarians are part of a religious community. The denominations do not matter, what matters is to be religious or spiritual. Church going has been shown to be associated with improved wellness and reduced deaths from all causes, compared to non-church goers.[144] Obesity, cardiovascular disease and cancer are reduced in people who attend a religious service on a weekly basis.[145]

Religious beliefs can shape communities, promote compassion and affect individual behavior. In the context of the Blue Zones, it is relatively easy to understand its beneficial effects on health, as it is part of a wider issue interlaced with community. It is more difficult to understand the immediate effects on health outside these areas. It has been suggested that those who are spiritual have less stress, as the stress can be relinquished to a higher power.[136,144]

Numerous studies indicate that religious involvement is associated with favorable health outcomes.[146] It is not yet clear whether this can be seen at the cellular level. There have been isolated reports looking at telomeres, which are a good indicator of cell aging. These support the theory that religious involvement is associated with healthier telomeres.[147]

LONELINESS

A growing number of elderly people are living longer and longer. Accompanied by this shift in demographics, is the specter of increasing loneliness and social isolation. This is a problem that has more bearing on health than you might think. Loneliness affects health as much as obesity and excess alcohol consumption.[148] The effect of loneliness on the health of people, who don't have a social network is the equivalent of smoking 15 cigarettes a day.[149] I always find the health statistics on loneliness both shocking and disturbing.

Loneliness affects all age groups from children to the elderly. Blue Zones have a commonality: people are involved in the community and have a sense of purpose. Loneliness is not found in the Blue Zones, and we know

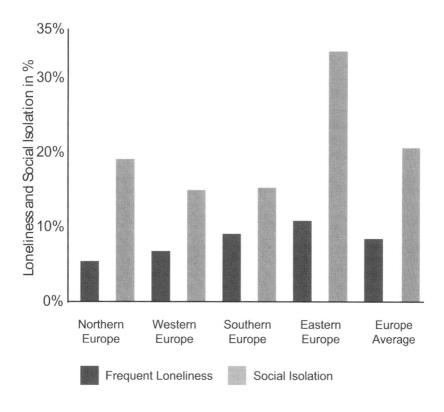

Figure 22.3. Regional patterns of frequent loneliness and social isolation.[150]

how healthy the inhabitants are. It is a fundamental prerequisite of health that social contact is maintained.

The EU spends its peoples' taxes on many things, including studying the population. The Joint Research center published data, as part of the European Social Brief, which showed that 7% of people in the EU are lonely. There is large variation in the distribution of this problem throughout Europe (figure 22.3).

This problem is so serious that some governments have commissioned campaigns to combat loneliness. Denmark has an active program. These include, 'Denmark eats together', which brings different generations and people with diverse cultures together during mealtimes. Hundreds of people take part. Social distancing enforced by COVID-19 aggravated loneliness.[151] Covid-19 reaped its damage in many unseen and indirect ways too. Public health campaigns need to do more to combat loneliness. We could all consider how we can make a difference to lonely people.

STRESS

Stress is a description of the surge of hormones and chemicals, which occur in response to a trigger. A stress reaction is a coping mechanism, essential for our survival. Stress allows us to deal with problems. We would not function without a well-developed stress reaction. We need the fight or flight response. This type of reaction happens so quickly that we are not aware it is happening. Our ancestors used it to flee saber-toothed tigers.

A stress reaction causes a cascade of changes in your body and your mind. This stress reaction allows you to react in ways you would not normally be able to do. It increases your performance, and you feel the changes; heart racing, focused instead of fearful. You feel powerful. You feel energized, excited and ready for action. Stress is energy. Athletes spend many hours in training learning to harness their stress response; in other words, use it to their advantage rather than suffer from it. Harnessing this stress response can make the difference between winning and losing.

Hormones are released during the stress response. They dictate the changes in your mind and body. Adrenaline and cortisol have widespread effects throughout your body. Adrenaline is the fast action response. Your heart rate and blood pressure rise. This pushes more blood to the muscles. Your breathing is quicker, supplying more oxygen to your muscles. Insulin is reduced, allowing stored fat and sugars to be released into the blood stream. The additional energy available to the muscles, allows you to run faster. If the stressful situation continues, phase two of the stress response is activated. This is a somewhat slower phase. Cortisol is released. Cortisol causes high blood sugar, high blood pressure and alters brain function. Your adaptation to the stressors continues.

After a stress reaction, you relax. You've escaped the tiger; you've run your race, and now you are safe. Another system takes over, and your heart rate slows, your blood pressure returns to normal and your breathing slows. Your body returns to normal and you feel normal. Stress is meant to be temporary.

But it can all go horribly wrong. If the stress reaction does not end, and you do not enter the relaxation phase, you are in a mess. Your body and mind remain in a permanent state of heightened alertness and preparedness. Your body cannot tolerate the prolonged surge of hormones and your long-term health is soon affected. The body stays revved up and is on high alert. We all know what that feels like. You can't sleep, you feel worried and anxious. Stress becomes a long-term problem. If the stress reaction does not dampen, the prolonged hormonal changes take a tremendous toll on your body.[152]

Persistently elevated cortisol results in elevation of your blood sugar, which remains high. Prolonged high blood sugar means insulin resistance. Your satiety centers are dimmed, and your appetite goes up. You eat more and gain weight. Weight gain increases the problem of high blood sugar and insulin resistance. You are on the road to diabetes. Cortisol raises your blood pressure, putting you on the road to a heart attack or stroke. Yes, stress can kill you.[153]

Chronic elevation of cortisol causes other health problems. Normally cortisol secretion has a circadian rhythm. There is a cortisol body clock. Cortisol is at its peak in the early morning; this helps you to get up in the morning and face the world. The cortisol circadian rhythm is lost in chronic stress. That's one of the reasons that stress affects your sleep pattern.

There are big individual differences in how people respond to stress. We intuitively know that people respond differently to similar experiences. Some people can deal with stress without any difficulties and quickly relax. These individual responses vary depending on life experiences, personality, social factors and genetic make-up. You can remain stressed for many reasons, including bad experiences in the past. Bad experiences in childhood seem to have a significant effect on poor resilience to stress in adulthood.[154]

Reducing Stress

A lot that can be done to reduce chronic stress reactions and protect your health. Not all solutions will work for everyone and people manage stress in different ways. But everyone can learn how to manage stress. People in Blue Zones encounter stress as well; we all do. They have daily stress relieving habits. These habits vary from person to person, from a happy hour, to a quiet nature walk or meditation. Find your stress reducing thing and make it a habit.

A healthy lifestyle with a good diet, regular exercise and getting plenty of sleep is the foundation of improving your reaction to stress. Sleep is critical to health and nourishing sleep will come if you have a bedtime routine. You should aim for seven hours sleep per night. Seven is the magic number. Attend to your sleep hygiene religiously.

Adding a poor diet to stress is stoking the cortisol fire with insulin. The two elevated hormones will together have a field day and cause havoc in your body. Cut out sugary foods and drink and stop the constant surges of hyper and hypoglycemia. Allow your body to physically settle, and the mental rest will come. Any exercise is better than none, just move a little more each day. Alcohol is not going to help resolve a problem with stress. It may seem like a good idea at the time, but in the long term it will prevent a recovery. Pills are not good; so, try to treat the problem with lifestyle changes.

Connect socially with others and share your problems. Loneliness will aggravate the situation. Engage with your loved ones, your friends and family. Socializing can be very supportive.

BURN OUT

A Burnt-Out Case, written by Graham Greene tells the story of Querry.[155] Querry is a world-renowned architect, in his mid 50s. He travels to a leper colony in Africa, run by nuns and priests. Famous for his church designs, he believes that the churches have been defiled by the occupants. He arrives incognito, trying to escape his past. He feels spiritually empty, with no emotion. He no longer enjoys life. Whatever fed his vocation, has ceased to exist.

Arriving in the leper colony, He is diagnosed as the mental equivalent of a "leper burnt out case", whereby a leper has gone through a mutilation and amputation, such as losing a toe. Querry slowly moves towards a cure, experiencing a rebirth of interest in life and humanity.

If you are exhausted, feeling detached and ineffective in your job - you may be burnt out. Burn out is a state of physical, emotional and mental exhaustion. Overwhelming emotional exhaustion affects all aspects of life. It leads to cynicism, and work is regarded as a burden. A feeling of a lack of personal accomplishment and a sense of ineffectiveness develop. There are different phases in burn out, ranging from tiredness and neglect of one's needs, through denial of problems, to depersonalization and the full-blown syndrome. Eventually ending up like Querry; A Burnt-Out Case.

Burn out is not stress, although stress may be a part of the problem. It is also separate from depression, although the two may co-exist.[156] Burn out may also occur with problems such as poor sleep and is a predictor of chronic diseases such as diabetes and heart disease.[157] Burn out can occur in any walk of life but tends to occur in professions working with clients or patients. It can also affect carers. It seems that doctors are particularly affected and there are increasing concerns about the mental state of doctors. Over 50% of US physicians are experiencing professional burn out, and the problem is worsening.[158] In the UK, there is an increasing trend for early retirement amongst General Practitioners and NHS consultants, which has been attributed, in part, to burn out. Losing senior doctors to burn out, will ultimately result in poorer patient care, and even more ironically, further burnout in the remaining doctors.

My sub-specialty area was diabetic eye disease. I tried everything to help to change unhealthy lifestyle in my patients. Sometimes with success, and unfortunately, sometimes not. I am reminded of this, thinking of one of my medical colleagues. She, of all people understood her problems and her risks and how she should live. But her eye disease was relentless and progressive. Intensive and regular treatment was preventing blindness but was ongoing. At a hospital social evening in the local curry house, I watched to see what she was eating. Naan bread, white rice and pakoras. I thought I was going to weep. It is this feeling of ineffectiveness, that contributes to burn out in every doctor, every healthcare practitioner, in every clinic. Every doctor is surrounded by the same stories, every day, every month and every year.

Worldwide, we face a huge burden of heart disease, diabetes, cancer and hypertension. These conditions are related to unhealthy lifestyle choices. Lifestyle choices, that we focus on in this book. Unhealthy lifestyle choices can be changed. The following scenario plays out on a weekly basis in our clinics: a patient develops adult onset diabetes, obesity and high blood pressure and goes to see their doctor. The doctor advises about lifestyle, the advice is ignored, the diabetes worsens, and the tablets are increased; still no lifestyle changes. The diabetes worsens, complications develop, more lifestyle advice is ignored; complications worsen, and it is downhill all the way. Blindness, amputations, and strokes follow. Multiply this story 100 times a week, 46 weeks per year and you can imagine that doctors will develop a sense of ineffectiveness, lack of accomplishment and cynicism. They burn out.

Five factors have been identified which increase burn out:

1. Long working hours.

2. Little downtime.

3. Surveillance by peers, superiors and customers.

4. Unfair treatment

5. Unmanageable workload

Whilst burn out is more likely in the health care field, it is something that you can face anywhere, regardless of your job.

No single measure will relieve burn out, but there are many approaches that combined will help. Individuals themselves need to change, but organizations need to adjust too. It is time to get together with your colleagues, time to share group experiences and for colleagues to extend support. It is time for superiors to engage and support changes within the organization. In

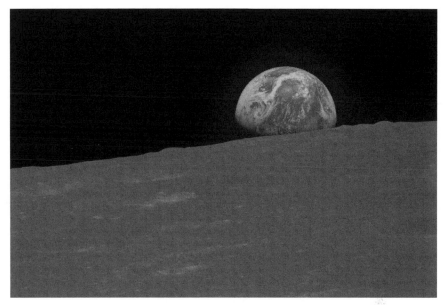

Figure 22.4. Earthrise. Apollo 8, December 24th, 1968. William Anders; "Oh my God, look at that picture over there! There's the earth coming up. Wow, that's pretty." Photograph courtesy of NASA.

hospitals in the UK and the US, this should be implemented immediately to prevent a future staff crisis.

On an individual level, there are many approaches which are believed to be of benefit. Relaxing activities such as yoga, meditation and exercise help to cope. Aim to sleep seven hours per night and pay attention to sleep hygiene. Work needs to be reframed with new priorities. Reach out to your friends, family and co-workers. If you are head of department, look after your subordinates, and monitor their behavior for signs of burnout. Socially, avoid negative people, and find new friends to expand your social network.

SLEEP

The crew of Apollo 8 saw the earth rising (figure 22.4). They knew, that although they had set out to explore the moon, they had discovered the earth. Earthrise, a photograph that changed the world, is celebrated as one of the most influential photographs ever. Anders was honored by the International

Astronomical Union, when they named one of the large craters in the photo "Ander's Earthrise". In Earthrise, we woke up to the beauty, loneliness and fragility of our planet.

Just like the earth, we sleep, we rise. Every day this happens. That's how life works. Life is dictated by rotation of the earth on its own axis. There is light, and there is dark, as we turn towards and away from the sun. The daily change in light gives life on earth its circadian rhythm. We adjust our lives, our bodies and our hormones on the basis of this natural rhythm. All life, animals, bugs and plants have circadian rhythm.

Circadian rhythm means that different things happen, as the day turns to night. During the day, there is building, energy expenditure and activity. At night, there is resting, repair and regeneration. Your body changes as the phases of the 24-hour cycle change. Your hormones, your nervous system and your gut bugs prepare your body and mind for the fluctuating activity levels.

You have a master clock in your brain. Local clocks are scattered in virtually every organ.[159] Your master clock keeps your local clocks in sync. Your master clock reacts to a change in light levels, with direct input from your eyes. It controls the production of hormones such as melatonin, which help you to sleep. Some local body clocks react not to light, but to other things such as temperature; but the master clock always has the upper hand.

Your synchronized body clock sets your circadian rhythm. Your circadian rhythm governs many biological functions. Animals, gut bugs and even plants have their own body clocks.[160] Your body clock controls the sleep-wake cycle, hormone release, eating habits and digestion, body temperature and other important bodily functions. Modern life has unsynchronized our body clocks. You can imagine that this doesn't do us any favors; our hormones go haywire, energy levels are affected, and sleep suffers.

We each have unique circadian rhythms. Some people are most alert in the morning others at night; so-called morning larks or night owls. Efforts to elucidate the reasons for these differences, have only now yielded results. We are starting to understand the mystery.[161] And the differences come from your genes. The makeup of our timing clocks is the key. There is a complex feedback loop in our body clocks. The feedback loop involves a protein called period, and an enzyme called CK1. A pause button, like the one on your TV remote, controls clock timing. The pause button can stop the clock short or let it run for longer. The pause button differs from person to person, due to variations in the makeup of period and CK1. If the clock runs short, we are larks, if it runs long, we are night owls.[159] If we have a fast clock, you like to do things early, if you have a slow clock, you like to do things later. And this depends on your pause button. Simples. Modern life, forcing us all into 9.00 to 5.00 patterns may be more harmful than we previously thought. Our body clocks also change with age.

An alteration of your circadian rhythm affects your body homeostasis. Hormones go out of sync. Hormonal disruption leads to disturbances of the sleep-wake cycle. Irregular circadian rhythms have been linked to many chronic health problems such as obesity, high blood pressure, diabetes, cancer and dementia.[162,163] Loss of the normal circadian rhythm is also associated with increased deaths, due to heart disease and strokes.[164]

People who are totally blind have no light input into their master clock. The master clock fails, and their circadian rhythm is no longer synchronized. They lack the necessary hormonal changes for sleep, such as melatonin and suffer chronic sleep deprivation.[165] I saw very few totally blind people during my career as an ophthalmologist. Of those that I did see, I can still see their faces, remember their names and their diseases. They had very sad outcomes from terrible conditions. Whilst deeply affected by the trauma of their disease, I have to confess that I did not appreciate how much their lives and health were affected by the effect of light deprivation on their body clock.[166]

Disturbances of circadian rhythm influences our entire bodies, by the effect on hormones, the effect on the gut bugs and all the other chemicals that control our bodies. A universal finding is that there is overaction of the sympathetic nervous system, in other words, a stress reaction. It causes many chemical changes, including inflammation.[167] Inflammation is something that you want to avoid for good health. If inflammation goes unchecked, you will not be looking, nor feeling your best for long.

Circadian rhythm is altered in jet lag, long-term shift workers and Monday morning blues. Do you struggle to get out of bed on Monday morning? If so, your Monday morning blues could be social jet lag. Changing your sleep pattern at the weekend, results in delayed circadian rhythm with fatigue and sleepiness on Monday. Shift work is linked to increased heart disease and death, from all causes. People pay a heavy price to keep hospitals open and the wheels of industry turning.

If you want perfect health, you need both the right quality sleep and the right amount of sleep. During sleep, your body processes go from active to resting. When you go to sleep, your heart rate and breathing slow and your muscles go limp. That's why, unlike most animals, you can't sleep in tree! During sleep, growth hormone, appears in high concentrations and repairs your muscles following the day's toil. Athletes are very aware of the importance of a good sleep habit, which allows their body to repair and subsequently improve performance. Sleep is so important to health that when we change our sleep even by an hour, we can see the direct effects.

Every year, many of us are subject to one of the biggest experiments in the world. And rightly, the controversy about this practice never abates. In spring every year, 75 countries in the world switch to daylight saving time. We add an hour of light to our evenings. The potential benefits include more time for outdoor exercise, using less artificial light in the evening and reducing road traffic accidents. But we lose an hour's sleep and our circadian rhythm is disrupted. This affects our health. In the week after the clocks spring forward, the number of fatal heart attacks go up. The risk of heart attack goes up by as much as 6% in the three days after spring daylight saving time. Deaths from other health problems, such as strokes, also rise.[168] We give away an hour's sleep at our peril.

Sleep is essential for brain health, particularly for tasks such as memory and learning.[169] Your brain is particularly active during certain phases of sleep. Sleep restores the brain and allows memory management. Data is transferred from your short-term memory storage area to your long-term area. During the day, the short-term storage fills up. At night, this data is transferred to long-term storage. Sleep clicks the save button on what you have learned during the day. The crowded short-term storage area then has room for the activities on the following day. But only in REM sleep. If you don't get enough REM sleep, your memories will not be saved. High quality sleep is a prerequisite for a healthy you, both for your brain and your body.

I remember chronic sleep deprivation only too well. Many months of chronic sleep deprivation followed qualification as a doctor, in the 1980s. We didn't have shifts, we worked our day job, then our night resident on-call, followed by our day job and so on. The most arduous rotas scheduled this every second night and every second weekend. We were chronically sleep deprived but young enough perhaps to survive it. One night when I was on call, I was woken up by a phone call asking me to come to intensive care urgently. I jumped up, sprinted to intensive care, expecting the worst. But it was all quiet. There was no emergency. The blank faces of the ICU nurses said it all. I wasn't the first and probably not the last young doctor to be confused. Nobody had phoned me. Perhaps it was a nightmare? Perhaps a hallucination?

We all know when we are not getting enough sleep, because our brains don't work as well as they usually do, our emotions may be labile, and we may accidentally fall asleep during the day. We can't remember things, and we all recognize the problems caused in our brains from sleep deprivation. However, few of us would normally consider what was happening in our bodies at the same time. If we don't sleep well, our bodies are under stress.

Sleep needs to be a routine, which means going to sleep and getting up at the same time every day. Seven hours sleep is the magic number.[170] Consistently sleeping between six and eight hours per night is optimal for health and no studies show that this amount of sleep is harmful. There is widespread agreement that if you sleep less than 6 hours per night, you are at risk of developing health problems.[162] There is some evidence that sleeping longer than eight hours is associated with disease risk, but there is less widespread agreement about this point.[171]

Naps are an interesting one. Many cultures, particularly those in hot climates have a long history of siestas. Ikarians, take an afternoon nap, as part of their downshift time. Ikarians live in a Blue Zone, one of the places in the world, where people stay healthy, live a long productive life, and forget to die.

A large study in Greece, evaluated the effect of siestas on heart disease. The population were all healthy at the start of the study. Over the course of six years, some people continued their siestas and some people stopped their siestas. At the end of the study, there was a large difference in the risk of developing heart disease between these groups. The siesta group fared much better than the group who did not have siestas.[172] Siestas of any kind were associated with a 34% lower risk of dying of heart disease, even accounting for other risk factors. However, a more recent study has shown the opposite.[173]

We cannot be certain about the effect of naps on health. Can the past give us some clues? No one can know whether our ancestors had a nap or not. People living in non-industrialized, traditional, isolated communities may be more representative of our past. The Hadza people may give us some clue. They have been found to nap, but nap infrequently.[174] In conclusion, we don't know definitively whether a nap is a good or a bad thing.

There are 4 phases of sleep, which include REM and non-REM sleep. You need to have a certain amount of each type of sleep for a nourishing sleep. Your seven hours of sleep matters, but it must be high quality sleep. Alcohol stops REM sleep. You may think that you have slept well after a night's drinking, but your brain waves show no REM sleep. You need REM sleep to learn, to create memories and to maintain pathways in your brain.

We can now monitor exactly what is going on with our fitness watches. We've all become sleep experts. The internet is awash with sleep advice and sleep apps. You can now work out yourself how different things affect your sleep. A consistent finding in sleep assessment, is that we sleep more that we think. You may have found this on your watch. You wake up tired in the morning, feeling that you did not sleep a wink. Awake all night. You look at your sleep data, you were awake for only 10 minutes. Scientists have uniformly documented that we usually underestimate the amount of sleep that we get.[175]

Sleep hygiene is the process of getting ready for sleep. Your body needs to be prepared for sleep. Women may be able to multitask, but our bodies cannot be in a state of rest and recovery and at the same time do active things. Develop a relaxing bedtime routine will work wonders for your sleep. Your circadian clocks can only change a little at a time, try to help them, choose a bedtime and try to stick to it. Alcohol may seem to help but due to its adverse effect on sleep quality, it is really not helping you. Sleep after alcohol, like sleeping pills, is a type of sedation and blocks REM sleep. We know that you need your REM sleep to save your memories from that day. Who knew that the tipple we had as students after a day's study was wiping the slate clean?

Electronic devices normally emit blue light, sending a wakening signal to your master clock. Most electronic devices now have a night setting, which is an absence of blue light. The yellow or night light does not send a wakening light to your master clock. However, a book and bedside lamp avoid all the problems of electronic devices. You need to practice sleep hygiene with your partner, or at least find the best compromise for both. You're hardly going to be settling down for the night, if they are doing a jig. As I can very well report, that's an issue when a lark lives with an owl.

It's important to exercise, but not at the expense of your sleep. Exercising raises your body temperature, which takes one to two hours to return to normal. Normally, our body clocks start to reduce our body temperature two hours before sleep. It is counterintuitive to raise your core temperature with exercise, immediately before sleep. You are fighting your hormones; they are saying cool down and you have made everything hot. Be warned, your hormones are going to win; they always do.

How to Sleep Better

- Go to bed and rise at the same time each day — develop a routine.

- Develop a bedtime routine.

- Exclude caffeine for at least 6 hours prior to bedtime, for some even longer.

- Finish your meals within four to six hours of bedtime.

- Make your bedroom conducive to sleep — dark, cool and no screens.

- Even a television screen that is switched off, is a big mistake.

- Don't exercise vigorously immediately before bed — try to finish at least 1-2 hours before bedtime.

- Birds of a feather stick together. Larks, live with larks; owls, live with owls

TELOMERES

What Is A Telomere and What Do They Do?

Telomeres are the protective tips at the ends of the chromosomes (figure 22.5). Telomeres protect your cells and without them, cells cannot survive.[154] They are composed of DNA. Your DNA pattern is unique to you. You can imagine that when scientists discovered that we all share the same DNA pattern in our telomeres, everyone was surprised. Telomeres have a sequence TTAGGG. This is repeated for the entire length of the telomere, hundreds and thousands of times. The 23 pairs of chromosomes are located in the cell nucleus and each chromosome has telomeres at both ends. The chromosome and telomeres are composed of DNA. DNA is grouped into genes within your chromosome.

The cells in our bodies continually replicate. That's the wonder of life. Some cells, such as blood cells replicate every few days. The fat cell turnover is the slowest, once every eight years. These are then replaced of course. Losing fat means losing fat from within our fat cells, not losing cells, which have a remarkably constant number throughout adult life. A few cells, such as nervous tissues cells do not replicate at all. Cell replication is a delicate operation, requiring the cell template, our DNA, to unravel. In the unraveled state our DNA is vulnerable, and the telomeres protect the DNA during this delicate phase of cell replication. telomeres protect this delicate unfolded DNA making cell replication safer.

Your telomeres pay the price for cell replication. By protecting the rest of

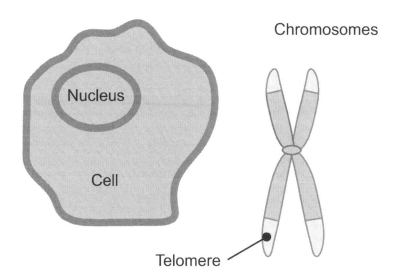

Figure 22.5. The 23 pairs of chromosomes are located in the cell nucleus. Each chromosome has telomeres at both ends. The chromosome and the telomeres are composed of DNA. DNA is grouped into genes within your chromosome.

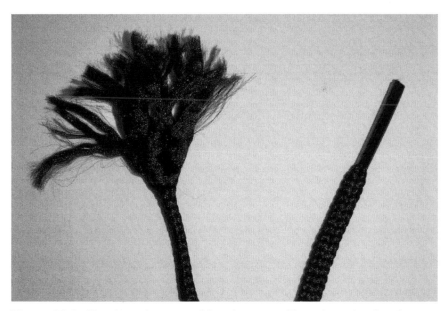

Figure 22.6. Shoelace tips resemble telomeres. If you lose the tips the shoelace will fray. Similarly, if you lose your telomeres, senescence, aging and cell death will follow.

the chromosome, they take one for the team, and end up shorter themselves. Every time your cells replicate, your telomeres shorten. Like a battle-weary soldier, the telomeres can only take so much. Eventually, they become so short, that they can no longer protect the chromosome, and the cell stops replicating. Cell renewal is now at an end and the cell starts to age. Shoelace tips resemble telomeres. If you lose the tips, the shoelace will fray, and similarly if you lose your telomeres, senescence, aging and cell death soon follow (figure 22.6).

Once the cell starts to age, it sends out distress signals. This is a process called senescence.[176] Unfortunately, the cell can stay like this, for a long time, even years. But it keeps sending out the distress signals. The distress signals cause inflammation, which spreads to other cells. Other adjoining cells then become senescent themselves. The accompanying inflammation spreads all around the body, causing "inflamaging", a combination of inflammation and aging. Senescence is one of the main drivers of aging and many long-term diseases.[177] Senescence drives the beginning of your diseasespan. And telomere shortening starts this process.

What Causes Telomere Shortening?

Telomeres shorten after each replication. telomere shortening can be accelerated by other factors. Free radicals damage and cause shortening of telomeres. Think of free radicals as waste products. Our bodies produce free radicals when we live, breathe and think. We actually need free radicals; they are a crucial part of immune system.[178] We live with a constantly low level of free radicals.

Free radicals can be pretty dangerous, as the name implies, but our bodies know how to hold them in check.[179] Our waste management system uses antioxidants to render free radicals harmless. In health, there is a balance between antioxidants and free radicals. If free radicals overwhelm the waste management system, a chain reaction develops. This cascade, called oxidative stress, shortens your telomeres. Oxidative stress develops from many stimuli including smoking, inflammatory food and drinks. The chain reaction damages cells and contributes to both aging, inflamaging and the development of many long-term diseases.

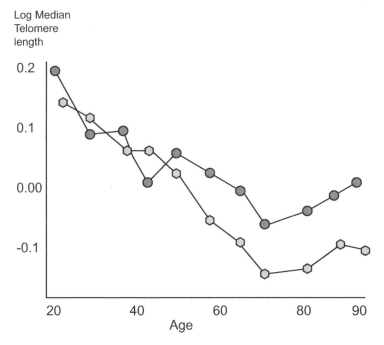

Figure 22.7. Telomeres shorten with age. The data shows a small reversal after age 75, which likely represents the survival of those who had longer telomeres from the start.

Oxidative stress plays a role in telomere shortening. A sedentary lifestyle, stress, poor diet, smoking and obesity all cause oxidative stress, which shortens telomeres. Conversely, exercise and stress management have been shown to increase telomerase and reduce telomere shortening and thereby protect from aging, senescence and cell death.

Your telomere length at birth is highly heritable.[180] There is a large variation in absolute telomere length between individuals, but all telomeres shorten with age. At birth, you have 10,000 repetitions of the TAGGG sequence per end chromosome; by the age of 65 years, you have only 4,800 repetitions. The older that you are, the shorter that your telomeres become.[181] After the age of 75, the people who are still alive are the ones who avoided accelerated telomere shortening or had longer telomeres all along (figure 22.7).

Does Telomere Length Matter?

Telomere length is a marker that determines overall health, lifespan and the rate of aging.[182,183] You can appreciate that telomere length does matter.[184] Short telomeres are consistently associated with increased death, from all causes. [185,186]

Telomere length is affected, not just by your age but also by your environment and lifestyle. People who live in Blue Zones have longer telomeres than people who live in other areas, of the same country.[187] And people who live in Blue Zones are largely free from long-term illnesses and obesity. They have long lifespans, long healthspans and short diseasespans.

The natural shortening of telomeres seen with increasing age, is accelerated in some people. Lifestyle factors increase the rate of telomere shortening. Short telomeres have been found in many diseases, including heart disease, high blood pressure, dementia, diabetes and cancer. Even worse, short telomeres have been identified as a marker of disease severity. The shorter the telomeres, the higher the likelihood of death from cancer. In some conditions, the shorter the telomeres, the more severe the disease.[182,188]

The Telomerase Story

The telomere story might have ended here, were it not for Professor Elizabeth Blackburn and her team.[154] The first to discover the molecular structure of telomeres, the first to discover the role of telomeres in cell replication, she then opened the door to the treatment of aging and disease. She discovered telomerase, an enzyme that can repair telomeres. She discovered that telomeres can lengthen. Fittingly, she was awarded the Nobel prize for Medicine.

Another Eureka moment! Telomere shortening can be slowed, prevented or reversed. And telomeres can be renewed. And the answer is not really that complicated. Provide the right environment, live the right life, and your body will naturally increase telomerase.

Accelerated telomere shortening can be reversed. You can change the accelerated downward trajectory. The right environment means creating a balance in your body and furthermore a balance in your life. Your mental state really affects your telomeres. Factors that shorten your telomeres include stress, depression, negativity, lack of exercise, smoking, poor diet, toxins, obesity, long-term diseases and poor sleep patterns. Let us consider some changes, that can improve the health of your telomeres.

How to Look After Your Telomeres

You may be surprised to find that stress shortens your telomeres.[154] Stress is one of the most constant predictors of short telomeres. Chronic stress can reduce the supply of telomerase. The type of stress determines how big the effect is. Early life stresses seem to have the largest effects, setting in place exaggerated responses throughout life that maintain short telomeres. It may be that stress in early life prevents learning how to deal with stress, in a helpful way. Life is stressful, we all have stresses. What affects our telomeres, is our response to stress and the way that it is handled. Taking measures to relieve stress, and alter our handling of stress, has been shown to reverse changes in the telomeres. Measures which have been shown to help include meditation, positive thinking and adopting coping mechanisms to stress.

Who would have thought that meditation could have a positive impact on your telomeres? Exercise provides stress relief and it may help to protect you from the damaging effect of stress on your telomeres. And keeping your telomeres healthy, slows your aging. Even positive thinking can help your telomeres. Stress should be approached as a positive challenge rather than a threat, and this is the type of mindset that will help your telomeres.

Exercise

Exercise keeps your telomeres healthy. Studies in twins have shown that the active twin had longer telomeres than the sedentary twin. Athletes have reduced telomere shortening compared to non-athletes.[189] Athletes also have higher levels of telomerase.[190]

You do not have to be a professional athlete to reap the benefits of exercise and to increase your telomerase. Triathlons are not required, and neither do you have to swim the channel. If you are sedentary, any increase in your movement is beneficial. If you are going to change your life from a sedentary one, to one which incorporates exercise, it is useful to know what you are aiming for. Ideally, the exercise needs to make you breathless. A useful target is to build up to 150 minutes per week.

There are three main types of exercise; long slow cardiovascular, high intensity and weight training. These all have different effects on telomeres. Cardiovascular and high intensity training have the biggest effect on increasing telomere length and telomerase. Weight training or resistance training does not appear to show similar telomere changes.[190,191] We all need to do weight training, as we age, to prevent age related muscle loss, but for your telomeres, cardiovascular activity is most effective. For optimum health, you need to combine all three.

Exercise improves telomere health by reducing free radical load. It is not just that exercise is good for you, but the corollary is true; a sedentary life is terrible for your health. Without exercise, your telomeres are shorter. The direct benefits of exercise help both your gut bugs and your telomeres; so, keep moving.

Food

What we eat affects our telomeres. Good foods reduce telomere shortening and bad foods accelerate telomere shortening. Super-refined carbohydrates, such as white bread, fruit juices and cakes, are inflammatory. They cause release of chemicals that cause inflammation. We have already learned that inflammation can damage your telomeres. Drinking 20 ounces (c. 1 pint) of sugary soda, every day is the equivalent of 4.6 years of aging, as measured by telomeres.[192]

Conversely, there are other foods that do not excite an inflammatory reaction and are anti-inflammatory. These do not cause telomere damage. Oily fish, rich in omega-3s, are anti-inflammatory, as are berries, vegetables, nuts, seeds and other plant foods. Plant foods contain natural antioxidants called polyphenols. These antioxidants will mitigate the bad effects of inflammatory food and help to protect your telomeres. Ideally, your diet should be made up of principally non-inflammatory or anti-inflammatory components, with a minimum of the bad stuff.

Research has borne this out. A high fiber diet is associated with healthy telomeres.[193] Eating a healthy diet of wholegrains, legumes, vegetables, fruits, seafood, nuts and olive oil is associated with longer telomeres compared to a diet of refined grains, processed meats and sweet drinks.[194] The American Heart Association recommend that people with heart disease take daily omega-3s, which improves their survival. People with heart disease, with high levels of omega-3 fatty acids, show that the rate of telomere shortening decreases.[195]

Weight

Weight is related to telomere length. A high BMI is associated with short telomeres.[182,196,197,198] Lean individuals have longer telomeres than people with normal weight, who have longer telomeres than obese people. The difference in telomere length between lean and obese people corresponds to 8.8 years of aging.[199]

There are different types of obesity and this makes the subject complex.[200] In obese people, the fat distribution affects the extent of associated health problems. The worst type of obesity is visceral fat. You recognize this easily, you will see some extreme examples at pub closing times, lots of people with fat bellies, overhanging tight belts and trousers. It's not called a beer belly for nothing.

Visceral fat increases the risk of diabetes, high blood pressure, high cholesterol, stroke, heart attacks, sleep apnea, cancer, gout, heart failure and arthritis. The list goes on. The least serious type of fat is fat under the skin, or subcutaneous fat. Obesity is associated with excess free radical formation or oxidative stress.[201] Oxidative stress in obesity shortens your telomeres.

Sumo wrestlers are, by anyone's standards, obese. Sumo wrestlers eat up to 7,500 calories per day, in two meals. Chanko nabe is the traditional dish, a stew, composed of protein and vegetables. Their exercise regime is punishing, rising at 5.00am, exercising for 6 hours. Keiko is not your average gym session, consisting of teppo (thrusting exercises) and shiko (leg stamps), repeated again and again. Sumo wrestlers can lose 6 kg in a morning's training session. Lunch is followed by a nap, followed by a further workout, followed by dinner and early night-time retirement. They do not have annual breaks in their unremitting physical routine and perform all year round. Sumo wrestling is a way of life and their lives are strictly controlled. They live in stables, led by stable masters, with a strict hierarchical structure.

Sumo wrestlers can weigh up to 330 pounds (c. 24 stone, 150 kg). But they rarely develop diabetes, high blood pressure, or heart disease. They maintain a healthy metabolism.[202] Scans have shown that their fat is subcutaneous, or under the skin. They do not have visceral fat. A FastSpan of 16 hours per day and the extreme exercise regime, seems to protect them.

Sadly, when sumo wrestlers retire, their metabolism changes. They rapidly develop high blood pressure, raised blood glucose and cholesterol, followed by diabetes and heart disease.[203,204] Normally retiring at the age of 30, they have a high mortality rate, dying at between 35 and 74 years of age. Similar findings have been found in other sports with large athletes, such as football players in the American NFL..[200,205]

The changing pattern of Western lifestyles has seen children becoming obese. Even childhood obesity, in children as young as eight, is associated with shorter telomeres. Those who have the highest BMI, have the shortest telomeres. Premature aging is now starting in childhood. Loss of telomeres is setting these children up for a lifetime of long-term diseases throughout adulthood. As telomere length predicts life expectancy, this may have serious consequences.[206] I use the word may, because we don't yet know what the future holds for these children or their telomeres, because the science of telomeres is too new to allow certainty at the present time. But it doesn't bode well.

But it is not all doom and gloom, as the situation can be reversed. The accelerated shortening can be slowed. Weight loss in obese people has been shown to lengthen telomeres in as little as six months, and if the weight loss is maintained, the difference in telomere length, at 12 months, is even greater.[207] This is one reason we emphasize the importance of permanent

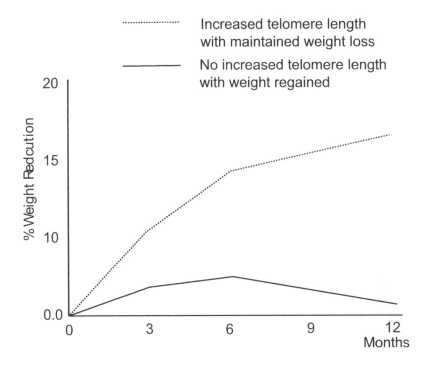

Figure 22.8. Telomere length in two groups, diuring a weight loss program. Telomere length increased in the group who maintained weight loss ar 6 and 12 months. In the group who did not maintain weight loss, there was no increase in telomere length. [207]

weight loss. A study of patients who underwent weight loss surgery showed telomere lengthening following surgery (figure 22.8). This shows the telomere length in two groups of people, during a weight loss program. telomere length increased in the group who maintained weight loss at 6 and 12 months. In the group who did not maintain weight loss, there was no increase in telomere length.

Paul and I haven't measured our telomeres. telomeres are difficult to measure accurately, and the world of commercial telomere measurement is largely unregulated. Also, telomere length is highly variable among individuals. The research into telomeres has been carried out using large numbers, where individual differences are smoothed out. What we are doing, is trying to do the best for our telomeres, without testing. At the present time, telomere science has not yet reached a level where it can be translated into personalized medicine.[209] This day may one day come.

STUFFOCATION

The concept of stuffocation was brought to the world by James Wallman.[9] He describes himself as a futurist, cultural commentator and experience strategist. He revealed to the world the growing sense of stuffocation. We have more stuff than we need; clothes we never wear, kit we don't use and toys we don't play with. This, he argues is making us feel stressed and in turn might be killing us. It struck a note with people, and the book was a best-seller. He elucidates that we should swap our worldly goods for experiences, live more meaningful lives and find truer happiness.

We spent two years decluttering our lives and feel very much the better for it. In our stables, we found five battery chargers; when over the years, I was unable to find a single one, was an embarrassing revelation. You may well have the equivalent of the multiple battery chargers in your life. While getting to this point required a big effort, we find that maintaining a decluttered life is both satisfying and easy. We have a strict rule now: one in, one out. It works every time; almost!

SKIN HUNGER

"What is the good life" is one of life's vexing questions. We know that happy couples have reduced cortisol levels, less stress and less disease.[211] Touch may be one of the big secrets. Humans are wired to be touched. We have a lifelong need for physical contact. We need it from the moment we are born to the moment we die. When we are touched, our brains can determine the precise nature of each contact, friend or foe, toxin or harmless element, genuine lover or lecherous slime ball.

Incredible emotional and physical health benefits come from touch. Increasingly, people believe that it is now fundamental to health. We can communicate compassion through touch alone.[212] A simple touch can release oxytocin, the love hormone. This makes you feel happy. Funny how you never see or hear of touch being suggested for health problems. We instinctively know that touching is beneficial; our modern-day language reflects this; "healing hands" or "feeling the love".

Skin hunger can have serious and long-lasting effects.[213] A study in preterm newborns showed that those babies who received massage gained more weight than those babies who were not touched.[214] In our new world of covid hysteria, where social distancing is the "new normal", and touching others socially unacceptable, we may well rue the loss of our brief social touches. At least with most people!

LITTLE THINGS MATTER TOO

Little things matter, both to your health and your wellness. You can live what you consider to be the perfect lifestyle; you exercise, you stay lean and neither drink nor smoke. You have a healthy diet and then suddenly, you develop diabetes. This could be related to your teeth. Studies have shown that the presence of poor dental hygiene increases the risk of diabetes and heart disease.[215,216] Gum disease allows bacteria to enter the blood, causing widespread inflammation. And inflammation plays an important role in the development of diabetes and heart disease. Conversely, good dental hygiene has been shown to independently reduce the risk of developing diabetes.[217,218]

Science is looking at other little things that may matter too. Eating dark chocolate in small amounts and infrequently may reduce your risk of heart disease and stroke. Listening to classical music may lower your blood pressure, getting out of the city may reduce your risk of heart disease, or having more orgasms (study done in men only) may reduce your risk of heart disease and death. So, if chocolate, music and country living don't tick your boxes — you know what to do.

It has been 37 years since I graduated from medical school. The day is etched forever in my memory. It was a sunny June day in Dublin. Six long grueling years of study were over. I remember a lot about that day, walking up to the podium to receive my certificate, in order of place in the class. Hierarchical results were not something that the university was shy of demonstrating. No wokeness in those days. It was one of the proudest days of my life and on a par with finishing my first Ironman triathlon in my 60th year. I remember who was there, where we went, even the dress that I wore. But I can't remember who gave a speech at my graduation, yet alone what was said. The graduates of the University of Texas, in Austin in May 2014 tell a different story. Admiral William H. McRaven delivered the commencement address. And this is what he said:

"If you make your bed every morning you will have accomplished the first task of the day. It will give you a small sense of pride, and it will encourage you to do another task and another and another. By the end of the day, that one task completed will have turned into many tasks completed. Making your bed will also reinforce the fact that little things in life matter. If you can't do the little things right, you will never do the big things right. And, if by chance you have a miserable day, you will come home to a bed that is made -- that you made -- and a made bed gives you encouragement that tomorrow will be better. If you want to change the world, start off by making your bed".[219]

The speech went viral, with over 10 million views. The phrase "Make your bed" is now a recognized mantra. A simple but profound message struck a chord with the world.

Wellness is an active process; different choices direct you to a healthy and fulfilling life. It is a dynamic, ever-changing process of change and growth. For Paul and me: It meant downsizing and leading a simpler life. It meant giving up our beloved careers in medicine and becoming prevention doctors. Our hope is that by reading this book, you will find true health and be able to maintain that health and that you will find wellness. You can make choices, armed with the knowledge that we have shared with you. You will be able to turn obesity around, prevent disease and share this knowledge with your friends and family.

CHAPTER WHISPERINGS

- The term lifespan, and its two parts, healthspan and diseasespan, focus our attention on what we are trying to achieve with wellness. We want to extend our healthspan so that we do not suffer long term diseases in the latter part of our lives. We want diseasespan to be as short as possible

- The people who live in Blue Zones share commonalities in their lives. Incorporating those common features into our own lives, can improve our wellness

- Meditation is associated with longer telomeres, an indication that the aging process is slowing

- Most people in the world identify with a religious group and this comes with health benefits

- Loneliness has terrible effects on your health which is the equivalent of smoking 15 cigarettes per day

- Stress is inevitable; what matters is you can identify it and learn how to deal with it

- Stress management can be learned

- Stress management includes a good sleep pattern, exercise, healthy diet, socialization, relying on friends, avoiding drugs and alcohol

- Burn out occurs in many professions, but is particularly prevalent in the health care field

- Sleep is essential for health

- Sleep induced by alcohol or pills, tends to be dream free, with less restoration and repair

- Disturbance of circadian rhythm has a terrible effect on your homeostasis and wellness

- Seven hours sleep is the minimum magic number

- You need a sleep routine to achieve healthy, restorative sleep

- You need to practice sleep hygiene, as a routine part of your sleep and get others to respect it

- Your body clocks control your circadian rhythms

- Morning larks have a shorter pause button in their body clocks than night owls

- Telomeres are the tips of your chromosomes

- Telomeres play a protective role in cell replication

- Telomeres shorten with each replication

- Telomeres can no longer protect the cell, when they reach a critical shortening and the cell then starts to die

- Senescence is the process of long slow cell death, which contributes to widespread inflammation

- Telomeres are a marker of aging

- Some changes make the natural telomere shortening accelerate; for example, obesity, stress, a sedentary lifestyle and a poor diet.

- Short telomeres are associated with many non-communicable diseases

- Lifestyle changes can lengthen telomeres and the trajectory of shortening slowed

- We all have too much stuff and this stuffocation contributes to the stresses in our lives

- Stuffocation should be swapped for life experiences

- Humans are tactile creatures and we need skin contact for health

- Little things in life matter, such as making your bed

- As coach Wooden says, "make every day your masterpiece"

CHAPTER 23

PUBLIC HEALTH AND BANKRUPTING THE WEST

"Rather go to bed without food, than rise in debt"

Benjamin Franklin

THE PROBLEM

Obesity will bankrupt the US by 2047, Australia by 2066 and the UK by 2086. I have modeled medical inflation with the average economic growth over the last ten years. Projecting these figures forwards we can see that the healthcare bill will reach 100% of GDP by these dates (figures 23.1 and 23.2). Well before these dates, the short-termism of our political cycles will have terrifying, yet predictable effects. An increase in demand for medical services will outstrip supply much earlier, as money is constrained; perhaps when health spend reaches 50% of GDP. Terrifyingly, in the US this will happen in 2035.

Doctors income will be forced downwards and combined with an intolerable workload will lead to increased burnout and early retirement. In the UK, hospital doctors average retirement age has dropped to 59 for the first time in history. Burnout is common when demand outstrips capacity, and patients have unrealistic expectations. During the corona pandemic, the "new normal" is not fear of a virus, but a failure to accept death as a consequence of life, risk and freedom. Many are now unable to appreciate the conceptual beauty of the finite. The real rose versus the plastic one.

As more doctors burnout and retire, healthcare quality will decline. And the cycle repeats. We are heading into uncomfortable times. Rational debate is prevented by mass hysteria, short political cycles and the new healthcare deity. Identity politics attempts to stifle open and necessary debate about

	2021	2035	2045	2055	2065
AUS	11.59%	22.67%	36.62%	59.16%	95.56%
UK	5.39%	10.08%	15.08%	24.66%	38.58%
US	22.16%	50.36%	90.51%	162.7%	292.4%

Figure 23.1. Mathematical model based on the last 10 years health spend and GDP growth. Health spend as a proportion of GDP up to 2065.

Health spend as % of GDP

	50%	100%
AUSTRALIA	2052	2066
UK	2071	2087
USA	2035	2047

Figure 23.2. Graph of health spend when it reaches 50% of GDP and 100% of GDP for Australia, UK and US. All data extrapolated from each country's health spend growth versus GDP growth over the last 10 years and avoiding 2008

obesity. I stress we cannot solve this problem by GDP growth. In the common parlance of this book, our economies can't outrun the obesity pandemic.

We have to stop the demand. Increased annual budgets should be for innovation and prevention; not more preventable disease management. Solve obesity and metabolic syndrome and the hospitals will be empty; just like they were in the non-covid areas during the pandemic.

THE CAUSE

Our diets changed 12,000 years ago, with the onset of agriculture and the first carbohydrate revolution. We learned how to cultivate wheat and then cleverly made delicious foods, such as bread, from these wild grasses. Over the last 100 years, our diets were transformed even more radically, as carbohydrates were used to make cakes, pastries and donuts; the second carbohydrate revolution. The introduction of refined carbohydrates followed by super-refined carbohydrates has adversely impacted our health. We have gone from creatures whose lives depended on food availability, to creatures where excess food is now killing us. The changes have happened too quickly to allow us to evolve and adapt. Some argue that we may have seen some adaptation to the first carbohydrate revolution, but it would be impossible for our bodies to have adapted to the fifty-times carb loading of the last 100 years. Our bodies cannot cope with the increased carbohydrate onslaught. We evolved over thousands to years to conserve energy; we had to, as food was scarce. In these modern times of plenty, we store too much energy and are becoming fatter and obese. We did not evolve to eat super-refined carbohydrates and our hormones, while perfectly designed to keep us healthy in the past, are now in a maelstrom of chaos.

We are at the mercy and whim of large corporate companies who fill our lives with adverts for foods we ill-need. We are awash with messages to eat more, eat three meals a day and then snack in-between. Such is the level of indoctrination, most people believe that missing a meal is a bad, or even worse, dangerous. Overeating and eating junk food, containing super-refined carbohydrates is the new normal. We are rewarded with sugar highs, a compulsive feeling that needs to be repeated again and again, and sadly, again and again. Our food environment has departed hugely from our ancestors, and our ancestral hormones find themselves in a perilous state, struggling to cope.

Our lifestyles, our communities and our working practices conspire to keep us sedentary. We move less than we did. People are socially isolated, and people are lonely. Antidepressants are rife, but we show scant regard to tryptophan in our diet, or for our microbiome's control over serotonin. We treat our microbiome like a weed patch rather than a beautiful cottage garden.

We have lost 20% of our sleep time in the recent past. We show indifference to sleep and the sleep hygiene that our partners and us need to ensure a good sleep cycle. Sleep is essential for our bodily repair, restoration and health.

We have beacons of light in the world, where people live to old age without modern disease. These Blue Zones are places where the environment is conducive to longevity and healthy living. People live in communities, have a purpose, and exercise is part of their lives. They practice religion, of whatever domination. People living in the Blue Zones enjoy long FastSpans and its advantages.

Our environmental, lifestyle and dietary changes have resulted in a pandemic of non-communicable diseases; metabolic syndrome, cancer, diabetes and cardiovascular disease and all their consequences. Rates of obesity are soaring and are not confined to high-income countries. Rising obesity is associated with poor metabolic health and a plethora of non-communicable diseases. But worryingly, even non-obese people are suffering poor metabolic health, followed by disease.

There is no single cause and no single cure to the pandemic of obesity and associated disease. Terrifyingly, even the non-obese are now developing metabolic syndrome. Our hospitals will be crammed to the rafters, stuffed full of obese people with obesity related diseases and full of people with metabolic abnormalities. The rest of us will have nowhere to go. That one time, when you may need some health care, you can bet-your-bottom dollar, you'll be at the back of the line. Your only chance will be if you can afford it, and if there are any doctors still standing.

PREVENTION, EDUCATION AND TAXES

- Publicly funded bodies, such as councils, the NHS and charities require a code of conduct to promote a healthy lifestyle, and lead by example. These organizations should lead a radical shake up of the whole philosophy of looking after their staff. In every new billion-dollar hospital, why is there never a staff gymnasium or health club? Why do we allow fast food outlets into our healthcare environment? What message does that send out to the public and our kids. The fact that many hospital staff are obese, shows the widespread lack of knowledge concerning the causes of obesity. These people, who are themselves fat fuel inhibited, are clueless to the causes of their own obesity. Insanely, these are the very same people advising our population on health, wellness and weight loss. It is time for governments to be bold. Time to stop the rot.

- This is not a trivial problem. To solve the problem, we all have to be prepared to change our mind set. Spending an endless stream of money on the treatment of completely preventable diseases, not only ensures a sick population, but is madness. If these are all preventable diseases, why not spend all new budgets on prevention? And tell people that the money is running out, and it's time for a national campaign of prevention. Ultimately, it will pay for itself. It's not idiotic public spending, it's wise public investing.

- The ideology should be one of prevention doctors, not cure doctors. We need to be brave and avoid group think. Identity politics must not prevent us debating obesity and metabolic syndrome. We must continue to debate the harms from metabolic syndrome, with obesity being its major cause. Moving forwards, we require a different approach based on the following;

- Public spending on the prevention of metabolic syndrome, is sensible public investment. It simply represents a wise and caring government, investing in its people

- Preventative and functional medicine; this should be a new medical undergraduate subject and post-graduate specialty; with a professorial appointment in every medical school

- Preventative and functional medicine needs a separate government ministry working with the department of health, and not for them. It must not be usurped by the power-hungry medical lobby and the money-hungry pharma lobby

- If necessary, governments may need to change their advisers. We need much more emphasis on prevention rather than cure. That shift should be a strategic ambition of a new cross-party group

- In the West, we have done really well in making it unacceptable to smoke. The positive intervention of governments to tax cigarettes to an unaffordable level has worked. Governments spent a fortune on campaigns to explain the diseases associated with smoking, and cleverly pointed people towards the benefits of cessation. They introduced plain packaging and banned advertising and sport sponsorship. And it worked. In the UK in 1948, 60% of the adult population smoked (female 41%; male 82%). The figure now is less than 15%. And we know that stopping smoking reduces cardiovascular risk by 80%. We now need the same level of commitment from governments to think outside the box on metabolic syndrome and obesity. If necessary, change their medical advisers and be brave

- To nudge people away from harmful eating, psychology teaches us that fear of future disease is not a great driver of change. Lung cancer pictures on cigarette packets did not significantly help the cause of stopping harm from cigarettes. This type of fear rises from teens up to mid-life then declines significantly. Real change comes from immediate reward through regained personal control. In real life, campaigns need to be skillfully created to emphasize the benefits of reducing weight and metabolic improvements. Negative fear mongering campaigns will influence some in their middle years but will be invisible to the under thirties

- We should invest in hospitals where functional medicine can be practiced; where newly diagnosed people with type 2 diabetes, can go to get their disease reversed by fasting, dietary and treatment changes. A sort of sugar and food detox clinic, where people with metabolic syndrome can have their hormones and lifestyle straightened out

- This is a public health matter; people don't choose to be fat. Babies are now fat. Toddlers are now fat and now some teens have type 2 diabetes

- Take super-refined carbohydrates seriously. They should be super-taxed to make them a very occasional and very expensive treat

- Trans fats should be banned forthwith. We are allowing take-a-ways and restaurants to feed our people with a substance we know to be a poison

- We should also consider a ban any foods containing HFCS

- All sugary, still and soda drinks should be licensed like alcohol and cigarettes and have a super-tax added, making them the same price as cigarettes. They are just as dangerous.

- All low-fat foods should be withdrawn from sale and banned if the fat has been replaced by any form of sugar substitute

- Commence a public awareness campaign on the major points above.

- Like cigarettes, ban advertising on foods with HFCS or those classified as super-refined carbohydrates

- Create a code of conduct for Government Funded Organizations

So, there you have it; not really that difficult to save the West in a few pages. Create government policy that favors intelligent public investment, over mind-numbingly stupid public spending, that is chasing its tail in a downward spiral of doom. And the people will understand this big and bold move from cure to prevention.

ACKNOWLEDGEMENTS

"You must be prepared to work always without applause"

Ernest Hemingway

The overwhelming devotion of scientists and fellow doctors made this book possible. Without their research and publications, we would not have the knowledge to tackle the obesity problem and develop the diet-whisperer plan. Doctors and scientists all from over the world have dedicated their lives to providing solutions to difficult problems. We are truly grateful. We also want to acknowledge patients who have shared their data and time, so that mankind may benefit.

A special thanks to Alex Baker of Uppso Ltd for helping with the production of the book and front cover. All the mistakes in this book are our own. Apologies in advance. We tried our best.

GLOSSARY

"These are but wild and whirling words"

Shakespeare; Hamlet

Aerobic Metabolism: Aerobic metabolism refers to metabolism which uses oxygen, compared to anaerobic metabolism which uses oxygen. Fat metabolism is exclusively aerobic and glucose metabolism can use either the aerobic or anaerobic pathway. Aerobic metabolism takes place in the mitochondria, the power houses of our cells.

Anabolism: Anabolism is a process of growth of new cells, maintenance of tissues and storage of energy for future use. It is a constructive type of metabolism.

Antioxidants: Antioxidants are chemical found in foods. There are hundreds of foods that can act as antioxidants. They fight free radicals in your body. Free radicals cause damage to cells and tissues and antioxidants keep them in check. Antioxidants are the equivalent of dousing water on the free radical fire. Your body does not store antioxidants and you need to eat them regularly. A billion-pound industry has grown up supplying antioxidants, but antioxidant supplements may not be as effective as food sources.

Atheroma: Atheroma is the term used to describe a build-up of material in arteries. This is also known as plaque and can accumulate over time. Deposition of abnormal material in the artery wall, leads to narrowing, or complete blockage of the artery. The material can also dislodge from the artery wall. Atheroma leads to heart attacks and strokes.

Atherosclerosis: Atherosclerosis is the condition caused by atheroma. See atheroma.

Adenosine diphosphate (ADP): Adenosine diphosphate is derived from ATP, when it has given up its energy.

Adenosine Triphosphate (ATP): Adenosine triphosphate is the molecule that carries energy within cells.

Anaerobic Metabolism: Anaerobic metabolism refers to metabolism which does not use oxygen, compared to aerobic metabolism which uses oxygen.

Autophagy: Autophagy is a clean-up operation. It is the body's way of removing damaged cells and replacing these old cells with new, healthier cells. It is a process of recycling and cleaning. Not just are cells themselves removed and replaced, but the structures within cells are removed and replaced. Toxic proteins are removed from within cells and proteins are recycled. While autophagy happens naturally, it can be triggered by fasting and a keto diet. Autophagy is a natural process, beneficial to your health.

Basal Metabolic Rate (BMR): Basal metabolic rate is the amount of energy which your body uses to maintain vital functions such as your breathing and staying warm. A formula measures your basal metabolic rate based on your age, height and weight. Your basal metabolic rate is measured in calories.

Your basal metabolic rate is determined by your sex, weight, height, age, ethnicity, body composition and genetic factors. You can alter and increase your basal metabolic rate in a number of ways. Activity increases basal metabolic rate.

Belly fat: Belly fat is a term that describes visceral fat. See visceral fat.

Bilateral: Bilateral means both sides i.e. both eyes.

Blue Zone: Blue zones are areas of the world where the inhabitants live the longest. The inhabitants demonstrate wellness for most of their lifetime. The people who live in Blue Zones have very low rates of long-term disease. They share commonalities of lifestyle.

Bioavailability: Bioavailability refers to the amount of a food or drug that is absorbed after eating. 100% bioavailability means that all the food or drug is absorbed and is able to have an active effect.

Body Mass Index (BMI): Body mass index is an indication of your body fat. It is based on your height and your weight. BMI tables give an indication whether you are underweight <18.5, normal 18.5 - 24.9, overweight 25.0 - 29.9 or obese >30. There are limitations to BMI as the formula cannot distinguish between fat and muscle. People who have a lot of muscle may appear to be overweight when looking at their BMI. The unit of measurement is kg/m2 .

Bowel: The bowel is part of your gut. It starts after the stomach and ends at your bottom. There is a small and large bowel, the small bowel located before the large bowel. There are in many names for the bowel, such is its importance to us. The commonest other names are intestine or colon.

Bug: A bug is a small organism. Bugs are too small to be seen with the naked eye. They can only be seen with a microscope, hence the other names — microorganism or microbe or the non-scientific name: bug. There are six major types, which include bacteria, viruses and fungi. They are everywhere. They live in the soil, in rocks, in plants and animals. They live on our skin and in our guts. They have adapted to every environment in the world — snow fields, boiling hot springs and even the Antarctic. You name it, you'll find them there. Microbial means relating to microbes, or microorganisms or bugs.

c.: Circa or an approximation.

Calorie density: Calorie density is the number of calories in a given weight of food. Foods have varying amounts of calories packed into them. For example, asparagus spears (five) have 20 calories per 100gms and chocolate 500 calories per 100gms. Foods that have a low-calorie density include vegetables, salads, fish, some fruit particularly berries and lean meat such as chicken. Foods that have a high calorie density include soda drinks, chips, condiments and sweets. See also nutrient density.

Calorie restriction: Calorie restriction is a long-term reduction of calories by 20-40%, where meal frequency is maintained.

Carb: see carbohydrate.

Carbohydrate (CHO): Carbohydrates are a macronutrient naturally found in food. There are three types of carbohydrates: sugars, starch and fiber. They are broken down in the body to release energy and typically form 50% of the calories of an average diet. They are an essential part of the diet, particularly fiber. Fiber is necessary to nourish gut bugs.

Carbohydrates are defined in many ways. A practical way of defining them is on the basis of the speed of digestion and subsequent absorption. Unrefined carbohydrates are slowly digested and are even essential for health and in simple terms are good. They include vegetables and legumes. Refined carbohydrates are broken down quickly and include pasta and bread. Super refined carbohydrates are carbohydrates, which are very quickly digested and in simple terms are bad. Examples of super refined carbohydrates are soda drinks and fruit juices. Regular consumption of refined and super refined carbohydrates is associated with health problems such as diabetes and obesity.

carb, carbs and CHO all mean carbohydrate.

Cardiovascular: Cardiovascular is a term referring to the circulatory system which comprises the heart and blood vessels. The circulatory system carries oxygen and nutrients to the tissues of the body and removes waste from them. Cardiovascular disease refers to conditions that affect the heart and blood vessels which include coronary artery disease, hypertension and atherosclerosis (=atheroma).

Catabolism: Catabolism is a process of energy provision for all cells. Cells break down stored carbohydrates and fat to release energy. It is a destructive type of metabolism.

Causation and correlation: Causation and correlation are terms used to describe associations between events. Events can go together — this is correlation, but this may not mean anything. Correlation of two events does not mean that one caused the other. It also does not mean that the two events are truly related to the other. It may be a spurious, chance finding. Causation is totally different. Causation means that one of the two events caused the other. But causation has to be proved and demonstrating correlation is not the same as proving causation. The mantra is this: "Correlation does not imply Causation".

There are millions of reports of correlation between two separate events in the medical literature. Most people confuse data showing correlation with causation. People assume causation, where none has been proved. Causation is more difficult to prove than correlation.

A study was published in one of the most prestigious medical journals showing that the higher a county's consumption of chocolate, the more Nobel laureates it spawns. The data is entirely factual, and the statistics convincing. The data proves a correlation between countries with high chocolate consumption and Nobel prizes. The data does not prove causation. But the headlines read: "Eating chocolate produces Nobel Prize Winners, says study"- Confectionery News. "Eating chocolate may help you win Nobel Prize" — CBS News. "Eat chocolate, win the Nobel Prize" — Reuters. Even the author of the study does not believe that if you eat more chocolate, you will have a greater chance of winning a Nobel prize. To prove causation, there has to be a scientific reason, which there isn't and the author, F Messerli said that 'the whole idea was absurd'.

CHO: See carbohydrate

Cells: A cell is the basic unit of living things. All living things are made of cells. A cell is the smallest unit which can be called life. We are composed of 30 trillion cells. Cells are the factories of our bodies. Cells make products that are used by surrounding cells. They receive oxygen and nutrients from the blood that flows around the neighborhood. Cells are surrounded by walls and the entrances are tightly controlled by hormones such as insulin. Within the cell, are numerous manufacturing rooms and multiple power houses, which make energy from imports. The center of the cell, or nucleus controls all operations, the secret code for this is stored in our genes.

Cholesterol: Cholesterol is a fat, which is found in food and also made in your body. You can make all the cholesterol that you need, in the liver from protein and carbohydrate. Cholesterol is an important building block for your body, forming cell walls and is used in the manufacture of hormones. Cholesterol travels round the body attached to protein carriers called low-density lipoproteins and high-density lipoproteins. Cholesterol is high in nutritious foods such as eggs, cheese, shellfish and meat. It is also found in non-nutritious foods such as fast food including deep-fried food, sweets and puddings.

Chromosome: A chromosome is a thread like structure found in the center (nucleus) of cells. Chromosomes carry unique genetic information. This information informs cells how to function and replicate. No-one shares the same genetic information (except for example twins). We have 23,000 chromosomes, which come in pairs. They are made of DNA.

Circadian: Circadian refers to the natural cycle of biological rhythms, which recur on a 24-hour basis.

Circadian rhythm: Circadian rhythms refer to the daily cycles of your mind, behavior and body that follow a daily 24-hour cycle. Body clocks control your circadian rhythm and the master clock is located deep in your brain. The master clock regulates the timing of your circadian rhythm. Treat it nicely, it will reward you.

Colon: See bowel

Correlation: See causation

Cortisol: Cortisol is a hormone. It is called the 'fight or flight' hormone due to its pivotal role in the stress response, a vital part of our coping mechanisms. It has widespread effects on metabolism throughout the body.

Dementia: Dementia is an overall term for different types of conditions. In dementia, three main things happen: memory declines, communication difficulties develop, and daily activities are adversely impacted. There are different types of dementia, Alzheimer's being one type of dementia.

Diabetes: Diabetes is a disease that occurs when your blood sugar is elevated. There is either a lack of insulin or resistance to insulin. In type 1 diabetes, there is insufficient insulin and in type 2 diabetes, insulin is no longer able to do its job. The causes of type 1 and type 2 of diabetes are very different. Type I means that the pancreas cannot produce insulin. It is a very serious condition, with no cure at present. It typically develops during childhood or early adulthood. Type 2 diabetes means that although there is plenty of insulin, it can no longer do its job. Cells have become resistant to insulin. The job of insulin is to open the cell gates and allow energy including sugar into the cells. Due to insulin resistance, insulin can no longer get enough sugar into the cells. Blood sugar increases in the blood and spills out into the urine. There is no such thing as a 'touch of diabetes' or a 'little sugar diabetes'. Diabetes is a full-blown metabolic catastrophe. Treatment is lifelong, although weight loss can bring complete remission of the disease. See also insulin resistance.

Diseasespan: The number of years that you live with long-term disease, before you die. Diseasespan is lengthening in industrialized high-income countries. People are developing long term diseases at a younger age and thus living for a longer time with these diseases.

DNA: DNA is short for deoxyribonucleic acid. DNA is the building block of our genes. All genes are composed of DNA. See genes.

EatSpan: EatSpan is the amount of time between your first meal of the day to your last meal.

Endocrine System: The endocrine system describes a system of glands, which secrete hormones directly into the blood.

Environment: Human environment is a broad term and includes matter and conditions in the surroundings which impact on the development, action or survival of humans. It refers to all influences on us that are not genetically determined. It is a term used in the debate of nature versus nurture.

Epidemic: An epidemic is a disease which spreads over a wide area and many people are affected at the same time. It is a term traditionally used to describe infections but is widely used to describe the spread of obesity.

Fasting: Fasting is achieved by ingesting no food or calorific drinks for a period of 12 hours or more. Intermittent or periodic fasting means periods of fasting, interspersed with periods of normal feeding. In this book, we use the term 'fasting' to denote both intermittent and periodic fasting.

FastSpan: FastSpan is the amount of time spent fasting, between your last meal and the next meal.

Fat: Fat is one of the three main macronutrients along with carbohydrates and proteins. Fat is essential to human life, and we all need fat in our diets. 60% our brains are composed of fat. It has many functions, it is a source of energy, it cushions and insulates our organs, it allows us to process the fat soluble vitamins (A,D,E and K), it makes food taste better, and it has numerous roles in metabolism, helping the heart and immune system. Fat is not the enemy that we have been led to believe. Some fats such as omega-3s are healthy fats. Trans fats are unhealthy fats, deadly fats in truth. There are five main types of fat: saturated, monounsaturated, polyunsaturated, cholesterol and trans fats also called partially hydrogenated fats. Foods like nuts, butter, cheese, oils, avocados and oily fish have lots of fat in them.

Fat Adaptation: Fat adaptation is the process by which we change our body from carbohydrate burning to fat burning. We change from using carbohydrate as a fuel to using fat as a fuel.

Fat Fuel Inhibition (FFI): Fat fuel inhibition is our inability to switch from using carbohydrate as a fuel, to using fat. Our bodies can use one of two main sources of energy — carbohydrates or fats. Those accustomed to do so, can change seamlessly from fueling with carbohydrates to fats and back again. Those who are not accustomed to using fat as a fuel, struggle to switch from carbohydrate fueling to fat fueling. There is good news, with fat adaptation, everyone can learn how to make the switch and use fat as a fuel.

Feces: waste matter remaining after food has been digested, discharged from the bowels; excrement.

Fiber: Fiber is a form of carbohydrate that the body can't digest. A sugary food, such as fruit, has both sugar and fiber and this slows the absorption of the sugar. This helps to protect your insulin stores. Fiber cannot be broken down into sugar molecules and it passes into the colon, in an undigested form. The undigested fiber then provides food for our gut bugs and bulk for poop. Fiber is also called roughage and is essential for health.

Free Radicals: These are chemicals that are highly unstable and reactive. Free radicals steal electrons from healthy chemicals, which damage these chemicals. Antioxidants stabilize free radicals and make them harmless. If we don't have enough antioxidants, free radicals damage our bodies, our cells and our DNA. Too many free radicals cause oxidative stress, which leads to long term diseases. Few things in life are all good or all bad and so it is with free radicals. Our bodies produce free radicals to help combat infections. We produce free radicals after exercise, eating or exposure to smoke, pollution and sunlight.

Fructose: Fructose is a sugar, part of the carbohydrate group of foods. Fructose is naturally found in fruit, honey and most root vegetables. It is a simple single unit sugar. It has the sweetest taste of all the sugars. Fructose is harvested from corn, sugar cane and sugar beet. This is made into high-fructose corn syrup. High fructose corn syrup is used in many processed and ultra-processed foods.

High Fructose Corn Syrup (HFCS): High fructose corn syrup is a sweetener, ubiquitously found in processed foods and drinks. It is made from corn (maize) starch and is a very cheap food ingredient. There are different concentrations depending on the ratio of fructose and glucose. e.g. HFCS55 contains 55% fructose and 45% glucose.

Homeostasis: Homeostasis means that our bodies are in equilibrium. The settings required are dynamic, responding to changes that we face. When the temperature changes, or we develop an infection, or our blood sugar goes up after a meal, our bodies adjust, to maintain a stable internal milieu. This is homeostasis. Hormones are largely responsible for controlling our homeostasis.

Hormones: Hormones are tiny chemical messengers. They are produced by the endocrine system, a system of glands that secrete hormones directly into the blood stream. Hormones bind to receptors and this allows the message to pass to the cell and stimulate the target cell or tissue to perform a certain action.

Hypertension: Hypertension is a medical term, used to describe high blood pressure.

Genes: Genes contain the instructions for your body looks and works. Genes are present in all living things. Your genes are passed down from your parents. They are made from chemicals called DNA. Each gene has instructions on how to make proteins. These proteins determine how each cell grows, works and controls different processes. Genetic is an adjective related to genes. If genes vary, we call this genetic variation. Genetics is the study of genes.

Genetic: See genes

Ghrelin: ghrelin is a hormone. ghrelin is termed the hunger hormone and is responsible to making us feel hungry.

Glucagon: Glucagon is a hormone. The actions are opposite to those of insulin. It signals to target cells to release glucose into the blood stream.

Glucose: Glucose is sugar, part of the carbohydrate group of foods. Glucose is the simplest of sugars, with only one unit of sugar. When we talk about blood sugar, we mean blood glucose, which is the same thing.

Gluconeogenesis: Gluconeogenesis is the formation of glucose by the liver from either fats or protein.

Gluten: Gluten is a family of proteins, found in plants. It is found in a variety of cereal grains, including wheat, barley and rye.

Glycogen: Glycogen is the storage form of glucose. It is composed of multiple glucose molecules linked together. Glycogen is found in the liver and muscles. Animals have glycogen as well. The plant equivalent of glycogen is starch.

Glycolysis: Glycolysis is the breakdown of glucose to produce energy

Glycogenolysis: Glycogenolysis is the breakdown of glycogen into glucose, which can then be used to produce energy

Glycogenesis: Glycogenesis is the formation of glycogen from glucose.

Glycemic Index (GI): The glycemic index of food is the value given on the basis of how quickly the food raises blood sugar. Sugar is the reference food with the highest glycemic index of 100. The score is divided into high (>70), medium (56-69) and low (55). Glycemic index is shortened to GI, which means the same thing.

Glycemic load (GL): The glycemic load takes in to account the amount of carbohydrate in a portion of food. Food is rated according to the glycemic index and the amount of carbohydrate in a portion of that food. Foods can have the same glycemic index but a different glycemic load. GL is considered high <20, medium 11-19 and low 10. Some high GI foods can have low GL scores such as watermelon, parsnip, banana and pineapple. This means that although the banana has the same GI as spaghetti, the glycemic load of one cup of banana (13) is less than one cup of spaghetti (25).

Gut: The gut is a long tube that runs from your mouth to your bottom. The tube is about 30 feet (c. 9 m) long. There are many names for this system-alimentary canal, bowels, digestive system, digestive tract, entrails, gastrointestinal system and intestine. The gut starts at the mouth, continues to the esophagus, stomach, small intestine, colon, and finishes at the rectum or bottom.

There are very tight defenses between the inside of the gut and your body. The inside of the gut is outside your body.

Healthspan: The number of years that you live without developing long term conditions. These include diseases such as high blood pressure, metabolic syndrome, diabetes, high cholesterol or cancer. People who live to a ripe old age of 100 years have long healthspans. They do not live with long term diseases for 20 years as many others do, as those people do not make it to 100. See diseasespan.

Hypo: See hypoglycemia

Hypoglycemia: Hypoglycemia occurs when your blood sugar drops below 4mm/l. It can develop in people with diabetes, if the balance between treatment, food or exercise is not quite right. It needs to be reversed quickly, as it can be dangerous, particularly if on treatment with insulin. Symptoms of hypoglycemia vary between people and include tiredness, hunger, trembling and sweating.

People who do not suffer from diabetes can also develop hypoglycemia, but not the dangerous type. Hypoglycemia happens if the body produces too much insulin after a sugary meal and blood sugar drops, an hour or two after eating.

Inflammation: Inflammation is the response by the body to an irritant. The irritant could be a bug or trauma or chemicals. Inflammation can be localized for example around a thorn in your finger or it can be generalized for example the cytokine response to coronavirus. Inflammation is mounted by your immune system to protect you. You need an effective inflammatory response to survive. However, your immune system can turn against you and create inflammation in so called auto-immune diseases, such as rheumatoid arthritis. Aging itself is accompanied by low level inflammation, a condition known as inflammaging. Low-grade inflammation has a role in the development of non-communicable diseases.

Inflammaging: See inflammation.

Insulin: Insulin is a hormone. It allows sugars, fats and proteins into the cells. Insulin provides the key to allow energy to pass into the cell. Without insulin, cells cannot be nourished, the cells starve, and we starve. You cannot live without insulin. Insulin is the fat controller. When insulin is on active patrol, all excess energy is directed to the fat stores. When the insulin patrol is finished, energy stores can be utilized, and fat broken down.

Insulin resistance: You are born with a certain amount of insulin. When you use that up, you are in trouble. Cells need energy and the energy has to enter the cell by crossing the cell wall. Insulin provides a key to the gate to allow energy to enter the cell. The insulin key opens the gate and allows glucose, protein and fats to enter the cells. Insulin keys wear out and become weaker. If you use your insulin keys a lot, perhaps you snack all day, or have a high sugar diet or you've doubled your size, you will eventually need two insulin keys to do the same job. A year later, you will need three insulin keys to do the same job. This is insulin resistance. You have worn out the insulin pony and further recruits are needed. The number of pony recruits is finite, and in spite of calling up the entire battalion of insulin ponies, you will reach the stage when you cannot get energy into your cells. You do not have enough insulin keys for your needs. You then develop diabetes. Insulin resistance is a precursor to diabetes.

Insulin sensitivity is the opposite of insulin resistance. As insulin resistance goes up, insulin sensitivity goes down and vice versa. Factors such as fasting increase insulin sensitivity and lower insulin resistance. Foods such as super-refined carbohydrates lower insulin sensitivity and increase insulin resistance.

Insulin sensitivity: See insulin resistance

Intestine: See bowel

-itis: -itis at the end of a word implies inflammation. E.g. appendicitis is an inflamed appendix

Ketones: Ketones are chemical substances that are made when fats are broken down for energy usage. They dissolve in water and cross into the brain, thus supplying it with energy. Ketones are also known as ketone bodies. Ketogenic means that the body is making ketones. You become ketogenic when you fast for prolonged periods or you follow a low carbohydrate diet. Ketotic is an adjective of ketones. E.g. A ketotic state develops after fasting.

Ketogenic: see ketones

Ketone bodies: see ketones

Ketotic: see ketones

High-density lipoprotein (HDL): High-density lipoprotein is the 'good cholesterol'. HDL carries cholesterol in the blood. It returns low-density lipoprotein to the liver for processing. It helps to lower the risk of heart disease, heart attacks and stroke. lipoproteins are produced in the liver.

Lean: Lean means the absence of body fat. A lean person looks strong and healthy. If someone is lean, they have high muscle mass and low body fat. It is different to a thin person, who has low body fat but very little muscle.

Leptin: Leptin is a hormone. Leptin is produced by fat cells. It is called the satiety hormone and has a role in suppressing appetite.

Lifespan: The number of years that you live.

Lifestyle choices: These choices refer to the choices that you make about how to live and behave. These are determined by your attitudes, tastes and values. Lifestyle choices include what you eat and drink, whether you exercise or not, how you manage stress, whether you smoke or not and whether you take drugs. Lifestyle choices have a major impact on both your current and future health.

Lipid: Lipid is another term for fat.

Low-density lipoproteins (LDL): Low-density lipoprotein is the bad cholesterol that collects in the wall of arteries. It is composed of fat and protein. LDL carries cholesterol in the blood. If your LDL is too high, you have a risk of developing heart disease, a heart attack or stroke. lipoproteins are produced in the liver.

Macronutrients: A macronutrient is a type of food which is required in large amounts in the diet. We typically refer to carbohydrates, fats and proteins as macronutrients. Water is usually considered to be a macronutrient although is provides no energy.

Metabolic: See metabolism. Adjective relating to the metabolism of a living thing

Metabolic Syndrome: Metabolic syndrome is a condition where the chemical milieu of the body deteriorate, heralding the development of more serious disease. Five factors develop: high blood pressure, high blood sugar, visceral fat, high triglyceride levels and low levels of good cholesterol or HDL. The presence of three or more of these factors means that you have metabolic syndrome. Like the obesity statistics, the statistics for metabolic syndrome are scary.

Metabolically Obese Normal Weight (MONW): The term metabolically obese normal weight refers to people who are defined as normal weight but show abnormalities of metabolism similar to obese people, with insulin resistance. People in this group have a higher than normal risk of developing metabolic syndrome, diabetes and other long-term conditions. The term metabolically unhealthy normal weight (MUNW) is used interchangeably with metabolically obese normal weight (MONW).

Metabolism: Our metabolism is a group of chemical reactions, that keep us alive. The reactions involve changing food into energy or using energy. Energy is used to carry out the functions of the cell. For example, if it is a muscle cell, the energy will be used to allow the muscle to contract. Metabolism allows the muscle to work. Thousands of metabolic reactions happen all the time in the body. Two main types of metabolic processes occur-anabolism and catabolism. Anabolism means that there is building up of body tissues and energy stores. Catabolism means that there is breakdown of body tissues and energy stores. Our metabolism is controlled by our hormones.

Microbe: See bug.

Microbial: See bug.

Microbiome: Microbiome is the term used for the bugs, which coexist with you. The term microbiome is used interchangeably with microbiota. According to the strict letter of the law, microbiome refers to the genetic makeup of the bugs and microbiota refers to the bugs.

Microbiota: Microbiota is the term used for the bugs, which live with you. They are present in your gut, called gut microbiota, on your skin then called skin microbiota. The term microbiota is used interchangeably with microbiome. According to the strict letter of the law, microbiota refers to the bugs and gut microbiome refers to the genetic makeup of the bugs.

Micronutrients: Micronutrients are foods needed in minuscule amounts but are essential for health. Examples include vitamins and minerals.

Microorganism: See bug

Mitochondria: Mitochondria are the powerhouses of the cell and make energy in the form of ATP. They are a type of organelles, lying within cells.

Mitophagy: Mitophagy is a form of autophagy which involves the mitochondria.

Monounsaturated Fats (MUFA): Monounsaturated fats are fats with a double bond in their chemical structure. Think of fat as a line of people, all facing one way. Two people in the line are holding hands, the other people are not. The two people holding hands represent one double bond, a monounsaturated fat. If more than two people are holding hands, there are multiple double bonds, and this represents a polyunsaturated fat. Monounsaturated fats are found in include olive oil, nuts, and avocados. Monounsaturated fat is a good healthy fat.

Morbidity: Morbidity refers to having a disease. It is also used to denote the amount of disease in a population.

Mortality: Mortality refers to the causes of death on a large scale. E.g. The falling mortality in Europe from coronavirus allowed relaxation of lock down measures.

Muscle Fibers: There are three main types of muscle fibers-slow twitch (ST), Fast twitch I (FT-I) and fast twitch II (FT-II). Slow twitch muscle fibers are resistant to fatigue and are our endurance muscle fibers.

Myelin and myelin sheath: The myelin sheath is the insulating cover around nerves.

Non-Communicable Diseases: Non-communicable diseases are non-infectious disease, which cannot be spread from person to person, unlike an infectious disease, which spreads from person to person. Noncommunicable diseases are responsible for 70% of all deaths worldwide. The commonest non-communicable diseases are heart disease, stroke, cancer and chronic lung disease. They are typically related to lifestyle choices which include lack of exercise, smoking and poor diet. Non communicable diseases are widely referred to as NCDs. The World Health Organization has a global action plan against these diseases, which is to reduce death by one third by 2030 through prevention and treatment.

Nature: Nature refers to the physical world, including plants, animals and the inherent characteristics.

Nature versus Nurture: The term; nature versus nurture is an age-old argument in medicine. In this case, nature refers to our genes and nurture refers to our environment. The argument is between those who believe that nature determines our individuality and those who believe that nurture determines our individuality. Of course, it may be a bit of both.

Nucleus: The nucleus is the brain of the cell. It sits in the middle of the cell. The nucleus contains all the chromosomes and genes of that cell. It directs all the cell action.

Nurture: Nurture is the action or process of caring and protecting someone.

It comes under the broad terms of environment. See nature versus nurture

Nutrient density: Nutrient density compares the number of nutrients to the calorific value of the weight of the food. As you start to eat less, it becomes more important to eat nutrient dense food, so that you meet all the requirements of your body. The most nutrient dense foods include kale, salmon, seaweed, garlic, shellfish, liver, eggs, blueberries and sardines. The least nutrient dense food is sugar, lots of calories and only one ingredient, sugar. Sugar is not an essential nutrient; we don't need sugar as we have lots of other sources of energy. There is no nutritional value to added sugar.

Obese: This is defined on the basis of BMI (Body mass index). Someone is obese if their body mass index is over 30 kg/m^2.

Obesity: see obese

Organelles: Organelles are specialized structures within a living cell. Mitochondria are examples of organelles; they are the powerhouse of cells.

Oxidative Stress: Oxidative stress is an imbalance between chemicals that are unstable (free radicals) and chemicals (antioxidants) that are stable, which neutralize unstable chemicals. If antioxidants outnumber free radicals, all is quiet on the western front. If free radicals overwhelm antioxidants, free radicals damage cells. An excess of free radicals causes widespread damage and inflammation, and this is called oxidative stress. Oxidative stress plays a role in the development of many diseases.

Overweight: This is defined on the basis of BMI (Body mass index). Someone is overweight if the body mass index is between 25 and 30 kg/m^2.

Pandemic: A pandemic is the worldwide spread of a disease.

Peak age: Peak age is a concept found in the oil industry. Peak oil is the theorized point in time when the maximum extraction of oil is reached. After this time, the rate of extraction enters a terminal decline. Peak age refers to the age that we are expected to live to, life expectancy has been rising. This rise in life expectancy has slowed, leading us to believe that life expectancy will start to fall, for the first time in modern history. Thus, peak age has been reached.

Polyphenol: Polyphenols are a beneficial plant chemical, that help to keep you healthy and protect against various diseases. Polyphenols are found in naturally in plants, such as red grapes, chocolate, fruits, vegetables, green tea, herbs and spices. They are natural antioxidants. Antioxidants neutralize free radicals. Excess free radicals damage cells and are implicated in many diseases. Our bodies should have a balance of antioxidants and free radicals to avoid inflammation, oxidative stress and long-term diseases. Polyphenols are available as supplements, although these supplements are likely to be less beneficial that real food.

Polyunsaturated Fats (PUFA): Polyunsaturated fats contain more than one double bond in their chemical structure. The best known are omega-3s and omega-6 fatty acids. They are essential for life. Your body can't make them, and they are critical for brain health. Polyunsaturated fats are found in oily fish, salmon, herring, mackerel, and sardines. These essential fats are anti-inflammatory and healthy.

Prebiotic: Prebiotics are non-digestible fiber compounds, part of the carbohydrate macronutrient group, that pass through our digestive system into the colon. Prebiotics are essential food for our gut bugs. They are fermented in the colon by the gut bugs.

Probiotic: Probiotics are live bacteria and yeasts, that are beneficial for health. They are found in fermented foods and pass into the intestine. Probiotics help to keep your gut bugs healthy.

Protein: Protein is one of the three main macronutrients along with carbohydrates and fats. It is found in both plant and animal sources. Protein makes up the building blocks of organs, muscles, skin and hormones. Your body needs protein to maintain and repair tissues. Protein is made up of amino acids, which are linked together to form protein.

Receptor: A receptor is a part of tissue, or part of the cell wall, which binds specifically to a specific chemical, such as a hormone. Once a hormone binds to a receptor, the hormone can than transfer a message to the cell and this triggers a certain action.

Refined Carbohydrates: See carbohydrates

Resveratrol: resveratrol is a plant compound, part of a group called polyphenols. You find it in the skin of red grapes, and some wines have resveratrol in reasonable amounts. Polyphenols are plant antioxidants. Antioxidants neutralize free radicals, chemicals that damage cells and are implicated in diseases. resveratrol is touted as being an anti-aging and disease fighting chemical. There may well be quite a difference in the health benefits of consuming resveratrol in food or drink, compared to tablets.

Sarcopenia: An onomatopoeic word describing our natural descent into frailty. Sarcopenia is the loss of muscle and strength. It is a word which sounds of death and it does herald our gradual physical decline. Starting in our early 30s, there is a progressive, inexorable loss of muscle tissue, which continues for the remainder of our lives. It can be countered successfully by a program of resistance exercises. Strength and muscle can be increased irrespective of age.

Saturated Fats: Saturated fats are a type of fat defined by their chemical structure. Saturated fats do not contain double bonds. Saturated fat is found in animals and plants including meat, butter cheese and coconut oil.

Senescence: Senescence means that a cell can no longer replicate. Most cells replicate, although they do this at different rates. Senescence refers to aging changes in cells.

Senescent: A cell is senescent when it can no longer replicate. A senescent cell deteriorates and shows aging changes.

Soda Drinks: Soda drinks are taken here to include carbonated sugary beverages, carbonated soda beverages, coke, cola, fizzy drinks, pop, soda, soft drinks, and soda pop. They may contain sugar or artificial sugar sweeteners or replacements. Soda drinks do not include alcoholic drinks and water.

Starvation: Starvation describes extreme forms of prolonged fasting, which can result in degeneration or death. There is long-term deficiency of nutrients, resulting in harm. It is completely different to intermittent fasting, where nutritional deficiencies do not occur.

Subcutaneous: Subcutaneous means under the skin.

Sucrose: Sucrose is table sugar. It is composed of one unit of glucose and one unit of fructose. Sucrose is a naturally occurring sugar, found in many plants-fruit, grain and vegetables. It is also added to many processed foods.

Super-refined Carbohydrates: see carbohydrates

Target Cells: Target cells are cells which have receptors for a specific hormone (or other chemical). The term is also used to describe target tissue and target organs.

Telomeres: Telomeres are protective tips at the ends of chromosomes. They are similar to the end of shoelaces. They are made of DNA. Their function is to protect the delicate strands of DNA during cell replication. They shorten with each cell replication. Once telomeres reach a critical shortening, they can no longer protect the cell. Replication can no longer continue. The cell then starts to age. Rather like the end of the shoelace, the shoelace begins to fray, and the cell begins to die.

Thin: A thin person is someone who has low body fat and also has low muscle mass. They are not strong, and it is not as healthy, as someone who is lean. Lean is someone who has low body fat and also high muscle mass; they are strong and healthy.

Trans Fats: These are killer, saturated fats and must be avoided. They are also called partially hydrogenated fats. They can be found in these types of foods; fried foods, margarine, vegetable shortening, baked goods and processed snack foods. Denmark led the way and banned trans fats in 2003. The World Health Organization has urged all countries to do likewise.

Triglycerides: Triglycerides are fats composed of three fatty acids, hence the name. Most of our fat stores are composed of triglycerides. When they are transported in the blood, they are attached to the same carrier protein as cholesterol. Good fats, bad fats and in-between fats all contain triglycerides.

Whole grains: Whole grains mean that the entire grain is present: bran, germ and endosperm. Whole grains are not refined. They include oats, barley, wheat, and rye. There are other whole grains, some of which do not contain gluten. Significant health benefits have been shown in people who eat whole grains. There are issues which include the high carbohydrate values and the presence of phytic acid, lectins, so called-antinutrients, that may reduce absorption of good micronutrients. They are not essential in the diet.

Vascular: Vascular is a term that refers to blood vessels. For example, "vascular disease" = blood vessel disease.

Visceral fat: Visceral fat, is fat which is stored within the abdomen. Visceral is the unseen fat, stored around your vital organs such as kidneys, liver, pancreas and intestines. It is not the fat underneath your skin. You cannot feel your visceral fat. It actively pushes out your waistline. Visceral fat acts as its own organ and is very active. It secretes hormones, usually the feminizing kind, hence man boobs in men with beer bellies. Visceral fat is very unhealthy. It is highly related to metabolic syndrome, diabetes, hypertension and heart disease. You can look thin and yet have a significant amount of visceral fat. You can estimate your visceral fat by the ratio of hip to waist measurements. Visceral fat can be accurately measured with scans. Visceral fat can also be called belly fat.

Unilateral: Unilateral means one-sided and bilateral means both sides.

Unsaturated Fats: Unsaturated fats have at least one double bond. They include monounsaturated and polyunsaturated fats. They are the good guys of the fat family.

REFERENCES

1. Mandini S, Conconi F, Mori E, et al. Walking and hypertension: greater reductions in subjects with higher baseline systolic blood pressure following six months of guided walking. PeerJ. 2018; 6(5).

2. Wheeler M, Dunstan D, Ellis K, et al. Effect of morning exercise with or without breaks in prolonged sitting on blood Pressure in older overweight/obese adults. Evidence for sex differences. Hypertension. 2019;73:859–867.

3. Most Obese Countries Population. (2020-02-17). http:worldpopulationreview.com/countries/most-obese-countries.

4. Daily Telegraph financial reports LGEN 2018.

5. Rubenstein AH. Obesity: a modern epidemic. Trans Am Clin Climatol Assoc 2005;116:103–113.

6. Pi-Sunyer X. The medical risks of obesity. Postgrad Med. 2009;121(6):21–33.

7. An, R., Yan, H., Shi, X., and Yang, Y. Childhood obesity and school absenteeism: a systematic review and meta-analysis. Obesity Reviews. 2017;18:1412– 1424.

8. Fitzgerald S, Hirby A, Murphy A, et al. Obesity, diet quality and absenteeism in a working population. Public Health Nutrition. 2016;19(18):3287-3295.

9. Wallman, J. 2014. Stuffocation; Living more with less. Penguin Books.

10. Peterson, J. 2018. 12 Rules for Life: An Antidote to Chaos. Toronto: Random House Canada.

11. Johnson R, Appel L, Brands M. Dietary sugar intake and cardiovascular health. A scientific statement from the American Heart Association. Circulation. 2009;120:1011–1020.

12. Lustig R. 2012. Fat Chance. Hudson Street Press.

13. Plomin R. 2018. Blueprint. Penguin.

14. Appel LJ, Sacks FM, Carey VJ, et al. Effects of Protein, Monounsaturated Fat, and Carbohydrate Intake on Blood Pressure and Serum Lipids: Results of the OmniHeart Randomized Trial. JAMA. 2005;294(19):2455–2464.

15. Pelkman C, Fishell V, Maddox D. Effects of moderate-fat (from

monounsaturated fat) and low-fat weight-loss diets on the serum lipid profile in overweight and obese men and women, The American Journal of Clinical Nutrition. 2004;79(2):204–212.

16. Esposito K, Marfella R, Ciotola M, et al. Effect of a Mediterranean-Style Diet on Endothelial Dysfunction and Markers of Vascular Inflammation in the Metabolic Syndrome: A Randomized Trial. JAMA. 2004;292(12):1440–1446.

17. Van Dijk S, Feskens E, Bos M et al. A saturated fatty acid–rich diet induces an obesity-linked proinflammatory gene expression profile in adipose tissue of subjects at risk of metabolic syndrome, The American Journal of Clinical Nutrition. 2009; 90(6):1656–1664.

18. Simopoulos A. The importance of the 6/3 ratio in cardiovascular disease. Expl Biol and Med. 2008;233(6).

19. DiNicolantonio JJ, O'Keefe JH. Importance of maintaining a low omega-6/omega-3 ratio for reducing inflammation. Open Heart. 2018;5(2)

20. Simopoulos AP. An Increase in the Omega-6/Omega-3 Fatty Acid Ratio Increases the Risk for Obesity. Nutrients. 2016;8(3):128.

21. Simopoulos AP. The importance of the ratio of omega-6/omega-3 essential fatty acids. Biomed Pharmacother. 2002;56(8):365-379.

22. Oddy WH, de Klerk NH, Kendall GE, Mihrshahi S, Peat JK. Ratio of omega-6 to omega-3 fatty acids and childhood asthma. J Asthma. 2004;41(3):319-326.

23. Bowden RG, Wilson RL, Beaujean AA. LDL particle size and number compared with LDL cholesterol and risk categorization in end-stage renal disease patients. J Nephrol. 2011;24(6):771-777.

24. Cruz-Jentoft A, Sayer A. Sarcopoenia. The Lancet. 2019;393:2636-2646.

25. Dupont FM, Vensel WH, Tanaka CK, et al. Deciphering the complexities of the wheat flour proteome using quantitative two-dimensional electrophoresis, three proteases and tandem mass spectrometry. Proteome Sci. 2011;9:10.

26. Manolis Kogevinas. Probable carcinogenicity of glyphosate. BMJ. 2019;365:l613.

27. Guyton KZ, Loomis D, Grosse Y, et al. International Agency for Research on Cancer Monograph Working Group, IARC, Lyon, France. Carcinogenicity of tetrachlorvinphos, parathion, malathion, diazinon, and glyphosate. Lancet

Oncol. 2015;16:490-1.

28. Gianbaneille E, Ferioli F, Kocaoglu B et al. A comparative study of bioactive compounds in primitive wheat populations from Italy, Turkey, Georgia, Bulgaria and Armenia. J Sci Food Agric. 2013;93(14):3490-501.

29. Dinu M, Whittaker A, Pagliai G et al. Ancient Wheat Species and Human Health: Biochemical and Clinical Implications. J Nutr Biochem. 2018;52:1-9.

30. Bordoni A, Danesi F, Di Nunzio M et al. Ancient wheat and health: a legend or the reality? A review on KAMUT khorasan wheat, International Journal of Food Sciences and Nutrition. 2017;68(3):278-286.

31. Geisslitz S, Longin F, Scherf K et al. Comparative Study on Gluten Protein Composition of Ancient (Einkorn, Emmer and Spelt) and Modern Wheat Species (Durum and Common Wheat). Foods. 2019;8:409.

32. Dhanavath S and Rao P. Nutritional and Nutraceutical Properties of Triticum dicoccum Wheat and its Health Benefits. J of Food Science. 2017;82:2243-2250.

33. Peter R. Shrewry Do ancient types of wheat have health benefits compared with modern bread wheat? J Cereal Sci. 2018;79:469–476.

34. Cooper R. Re-discovering ancient wheat varieties as functional foods. Journal of Traditional and Complementary Medicine 2015;5:138-143.

35. Gianfrani C et al. Extensive in vitro digestion markedly reduces the immune toxicity of Triticum monococcum wheat: Implication for celiac disease. Mo Nutr. Food Res. 2015;00:1–11.

36. Spisni E, Imbesi V, Giovanardi E, et al. Differential Physiological Response Elicited by Ancient and Heritage Wheat Cultivars Compared to Modern Ones. Nutrients. 2019;11(12):2879.

37. Schalk, Kathrin & Lang, Christina & Wieser, Herbert & Koehler, Peter & Scherf, Katharina. (2017). Quantitation of the immunodominant 33-mer peptide from ?-gliadin in wheat flours by liquid chromatography tandem mass spectrometry. Scientific Reports. 7. 45092.10.1038/srep45092.

38. Zevallos V, Raker V, Tenzer S et al. Nutritional Wheat Amylase-Trypsin Inhibitors Promote Intestinal Inflammation via Activation of Myeloid Cells. Gastroenterology. 2017;152:1100–1113.

39. Lachman J, Orsak M, Pivec V, Jiru K. Antioxidant activity of grain of

einkorn (Triticum monococcum L.), emmer (Triticum dicoccum Schuebl [Schrank]) and spring wheat (Triticum aestivum L.) varieties. Plant Soil Environ. 2012;58:15–21.

40. Tye-Din JA, Galipeau HJ and Agardh D. Celiac Disease: A Review of Current Concepts in Pathogenesis, Prevention, and Novel Therapies. Front. Pediatr. 2018;6:350.

41. Cianferoni A. Wheat Allergy: Diagnosis and Management. J Asthma Allergy. 2016;9:13-25.

42. Igbinedion S, Ansari J, Vasikaran A et al. Non-celiac gluten sensitivity. All wheat attack is not celiac. World J Gastroenterol. 2017;28(40): 7201-7210.

43. Kucek L, Veenstra L, Amnuaycheewa P et al. A Grounded Guide to Gluten: How Modern Genotypes and Processing Impact Wheat Sensitivity. Comprehensive Reviews in Food Science and Food Safety. 2015;14:285-302.

44. Costabile A, Santarelli S, Claus S, et al. Effect of breadmaking process on in vitro gut microbiota parameters in irritable bowel syndrome. PLoS One. 2014;9(10).

45. Lerner A, O'Bryan T and Matthias T. Navigating the Gluten-Free Boom: The Dark Side of Gluten Free Diet 2019;7:414.

46. García-Molina MD, Giménez MJ, Sánchez-León S, Barro F. Gluten Free Wheat: Are We There? Nutrients. 2019;11(3):487.

47. Sender R, Fuchs S, Milo R (2016) Revised Estimates for the Number of Human and Bacteria Cells in the Body. PLoS Biol 14(8).

48. Lloyd-Price J, Abu-Ali G and Huttenhower C. The healthy human microbiome Genome Medicine. 2016;8:51.

49. Gregory P. Donaldson, S. Melanie Lee, and Sarkis K. Mazmanian. Gut biogeography of the bacterial microbiota. Nat Rev Microbiol. 2016;14(1):20–32

50. Dieterich W, Schink M, Zopf Y. Microbiota in the Gastrointestinal Tract. Med Sci (Basel). 2018;6(4):116.

51. Turnbaugh, P, Ley R, Hamady, M. et al. The Human Microbiome Project. Nature 2007;449;804–810.

52. Integrative HMP (iHMP) Research Network Consortium. The Integrative Human Microbiome Project. Nature. 2019;569(7758):641–648.

53. Bilen M, Dufour JC, Lagier JC, et al. The contribution of culturomics to the repertoire of isolated human bacterial and archaeal species. Microbiome. 2018;6(1):94.

54. Almeida, A., Mitchell, A.L., Boland, M. et al. A new genomic blueprint of the human gut microbiota. Nature. 2019;568:499–504.

55. Moore RE, Townsend SD. Temporal development of the infant gut microbiome. Open Biol. 2019;9:190128.

56. Kim S, Jazwinski SM. The Gut Microbiota and Healthy Aging: A Mini-Review. Gerontology. 2018;64(6):513–520.

57. Schloissnig S, Arumugam M, Sunagawa S, et al. Genomic variation landscape of the human gut microbiome. Nature. 2013;493(7430):45–50.

58. Valdes Ana M, Walter Jens, Segal Eran, Spector Tim D. Role of the gut microbiota in nutrition and health. BMJ. 2018;361:k2179

59. Tierney B, Yang Z, Luber J, et al. The Landscape of Genetic Content in the Gut and Oral Human Microbiome. Cell Host Microbe. 2019;26(2):283–295.

60. Rea K, Dinan TG, Cryan JF. Gut Microbiota: A Perspective for Psychiatrists. Neuropsychobiology. 2020;79(1):50–62.

61. Cryan JF, de Wit H. The gut microbiome in psychopharmacology and psychiatry. Psychopharmacology (Berl). 2019;236(5):1407–1409.

62. Cryan JF, O'Riordan KJ, Cowan CSM, et al. The Microbiota-Gut-Brain Axis. Physiol Rev. 2019;99(4):1877–2013.

63. Yano J, Yu K, Donaldson G, et al. Indigenous bacteria from the gut microbiota regulate host serotonin biosynthesis [published correction appear in Cell. 2015 Sep 24;163:258]. Cell. 2015;161(2):264–276.

64. Agus A, Planchais J, Sokol H. Gut Microbiota Regulation of Tryptophan Metabolism in Health and Disease. Cell Host Microbe. 2018;23(6):716–724

65. Rooks MG, Garrett WS. Gut microbiota, metabolites and host immunity. Na Rev Immunol. 2016;16(6):341–352.

66. Schnorr SL, Candela M, Rampelli S, et al. Gut microbiome of the Hadza hunter-gatherers. Nat Commun. 2014;5:3654.

67. Spector T. 2015. The Diet Myth. The Real Science behind what we eat. Weidenfeld & Nicolson.

68. Oliphant, K, Allen-Vercoe, E. Macronutrient metabolism by the human gut microbiome: major fermentation by-products and their impact on host health. Microbiome 2019;7:91.

69. LeBlanc JG, Chain F, Martín R et al. Beneficial effects on host energy metabolism of short-chain fatty acids and vitamins produced by commensal and probiotic bacteria. Microb Cell Fact. 2017;16(1):79.

70. Martens JH, Barg H, Warren MJ, Jahn D. Microbial production of vitamin B12. Appl Microbiol Biotechnol. 2002;58(3):275–285.

71. Sommer, F, Anderson, J, Bharti, R. et al. The resilience of the intestinal microbiota influences health and disease. Nat Rev Microbiol 2017;15;630–638.

72. Thaiss CA, Zeevi D, Levy M, Segal E, Elinav E. A day in the life of the meta-organism: diurnal rhythms of the intestinal microbiome and its host. Gut Microbes. 2015;6(2):137–142.

73. Murakami M and Tognini P. The Circadian Clock as an Essential Molecular Link Between Host Physiology and Microorganisms. Front. Cell. Infect. Microbiol. 2020;9:469.

74. Kaczmarek JL, Thompson SV, Holscher HD. Complex interactions of circadian rhythms, eating behaviours, and the gastrointestinal microbiota and their potential impact on health. Nutr Rev. 2017;75(9):673–682.

75. Thaiss CA, Zeevi D, Levy M. et al. Transkingdom control of microbiota diurnal oscillations promotes metabolic homeostasis. Cell 2014; 159; 514-29.

76. Carding S, Verbeke K, Vipond DT, Corfe BM, Owen LJ. Dysbiosis of the gut microbiota in disease. Microb Ecol Health Dis. 2015;26:26191.

77. Cani PD. Human gut microbiome: hopes, threats and promises. Gut 2018;67:1716–1725.

78. Castaner O, Goday A, Park YM, et al. The Gut Microbiome Profile in Obesity: A Systematic Review. Int J Endocrinol. 2018;2018:4095789.

79. Le Chatelier E, Nielsen T, Qin, J. et al. Richness of human gut microbiome correlates with metabolic markers. Nature 500;2013:541–546 .

80. Ge L, Sadeghirad B, Ball GDC, et al. Comparison of dietary macronutrient patterns of 14 popular named dietary programmes for weight and cardiovascular risk factor reduction in adults: systematic review and network meta-analysis of randomised trials. BMJ. 2020;369:m696.

81. Dao MC, Everard A, Aron-Wisnewsky J, et al. Akkermansia muciniphila and improved metabolic health during a dietary intervention in obesity: relationship with gut microbiome richness and ecology. Gut. 2016;65(3):426–436.

82. Remely M, Tesar I, Hippe B, et al. Gut microbiota composition correlates with changes in body fat content due to weight loss. Beneficial Microbes. 2015;6(4):431-439.

83. Lacobucci G. NHS prescribed record number of antidepressants last year BMJ. 2019;364:1508.

84. Kelly JR, Keane VO, Cryan JF, Clarke G, Dinan TG. Mood and Microbes: Gut to Brain Communication in Depression. Gastroenterol Clin North Am. 2019;48(3):389–405.

85. Francis HM, Stevenson RJ, Chambers JR, Gupta D, Newey B, Lim CK (2019) A brief diet intervention can reduce symptoms of depression in young adults - A randomised controlled trial. PLoS ONE 14(10).

86. O'Keefe SJ, Li JV and Lahti L. Fat, fibre and cancer risk in African Americans and rural Africans. Nat Commun 2015; 6: 6342.

87. Stephen, Alison & Champ, Martine & Cloran et al. Dietary fibre in Europe: current state of knowledge on definitions, sources, recommendations, intake and relationships to health. Nutrition Research Reviews. 2017;30:1-42.

88. Yatsunenko T, Rey FE, Manary MJ, et al. Human gut microbiome viewed across age and geography. Nature. 2012;486(7402):222–227.

89. Vangay P, Johnson AJ, Ward TL, et al. US Immigration Westernizes the Human Gut Microbiome. Cell. 2018;175(4):962–972.

90. McBurney M, Davis C, Fraser CM et al., Establishing What Constitutes a Healthy Human Gut Microbiome: State of the Science, Regulatory Considerations, and Future Directions, The Journal of Nutrition, 2019;149(11):1882–1895.

91. Carey HV, Assadi-Porter FM. The Hibernator Microbiome: Host-Bacterial Interactions in an Extreme Nutritional Symbiosis. Annu Rev Nutr. 2017;37:477–500.

92. Remely M et al. Wiener klinische Wochenschrift. 2015;127:394-398

93. Özkul C, Yalınay M, Karakan T. Islamic fasting leads to an increased abundance of Akkermansia muciniphila and Bacteroides fragilis group:

A preliminary study on intermittent fasting. Turk J Gastroenterol 2019; 30(12):1030-5.

94. Stockman MC, Thomas D, Burke J, Apovian CM. Intermittent Fasting: Is the Wait Worth the Weight?. Curr Obes Rep. 2018;7(2):172–185

95. Bastani A, Rajabi S, Kianimarkani F. The Effects of fasting during Ramadan. Neurology International. 2017;9:7043

96. Zarrinpar A, Chaix A, Panda S. Daily Eating Patterns and Their Impact on Health and Disease. Trends Endocrinol Metab. 2016;27(2):69–83.

97. Paoli A, Tinsley G, Bianco A, Moro T. The Influence of Meal Frequency and Timing on Health in Humans: The Role of Fasting. Nutrients. 2019;11(4):719.

98. Pollan M. Some of My Best Friends Are Germs. The New York Times. May 19.2013 (experts don't take prebiotic supplements).

99. Cole G, Frautschy S. DHA may prevent age-related dementia. J Nutr. 2010;140(4):869-874.

100. Araújo J, Cai J, and Stevens J. Prevalence of optimum metabolic health in adults; National Survey 2009-16. J Metabolic Syndrome and Related Disorders. 17(1);46-52.

101. Ruderman NB, Schneider SH and Berchtold P. The "metabolically-obese," normal-weight individual. Am J Clin Nutr 1981; 34:1617-21.

102. St-Onge MP, Janssen I, Heymsfield SB. Metabolic syndrome in normal-weight Americans: new definition of the metabolically obese, normal-weight individual. Diabetes Care. 2004;27(9):2222-2228.

103. Joana Araújo, Jianwen Cai, June Stevens. Prevalence of Optimal Metabolic Health in American Adults: National Health and Nutrition Examination Survey 2009–2016. Metabolic Syndrome and Related Disorders, 2018.

104. Bradshaw PT, Monda KL, Stevens J. Metabolic syndrome in healthy obese, overweight, and normal weight individuals: the Atherosclerosis Risk in Communities Study. Obesity (Silver Spring). 2013;21(1):203-209.

105. Lee, J., Lee, J., Lee, J. et al. Visceral fat obesity is highly associated with primary gout in a metabolically obese but normal weighted population: a case control study. Arthritis Res Ther. 2015;17:79.

106. Shen W, Punyanitya M, Chen J, et al. Waist circumference correlates with metabolic syndrome indicators better than percentage fat. Obesity (Silver

Spring). 2006;14(4):727-736.

107. Kaur J. A comprehensive review on metabolic syndrome [retracted in: Cardiol Res Pract. 2019 Jan 31;2019:4301528]. Cardiol Res Pract. 2014;2014:943162.

108. Flint A, Rexrode K, Hu F, Glynn R et al. Body mass index, waist circumference, and risk of coronary heart disease: a prospective study among men and women. Obes Res Clin Pract. 2010 Jul;4(3):e171-e181.

109. Lee, K.R., Seo, M.H., Do Han, K. et al. Waist circumference and risk of 23 site-specific cancers: a population-based cohort study of Korean adults. Br J Cancer. 2018;119:1018–1027.

110. Flegal K, Kit B, Orpana H, Graubard B. Association of all-cause mortality with overweight and obesity using standard body mass index categories: a systematic review and meta-analysis. JAMA. 2013 Jan 2;309(1):71-82.

111. Kenneth A, Schatzkin A, Harris T et al. Overweight, Obesity, and Mortality in a Large Prospective Cohort of Persons 50 to 71 Years Old. N Engl J Med 2006; 355:763-778

112. Arnlöv J, Sundström J, Ingelsson E, Lind L. Impact of BMI and the metabolic syndrome on the risk of diabetes in middle-aged men. Diabetes Care. 2011;34(1):61-65.

113. Aucouturier J, Meyer M, Thivel D et al. Arch Pediatr Adolesc Med. 2009 Sep; 163(9):826-31.

114. Chang, CY., Ke, DS., Chen, JY., Essential fatty acids and human brain Acta Neurol Taiwan, 009 Dec;18(4):231-41.

115. Fitzgerald M. Run stronger and faster by training slower; 80/20 running. 2014 New American Library; Penguin.

116. House, S., Johnston, S., Jornet, K. Training for the uphill runner, Patagonia Works. 2019.

117. Carnazes D. 2006. Ultramarathon Man, Confessions of a Midnight Runner. Penguin.

118. Rudnicki M, Abdifarkosh G, Nwadozi E, et al. Endothelial-specific FoxO1 depletion prevents obesity-related disorders by increasing vascular metabolism and growth. eLife, 2018; 7

119. Yerushalmy J, Hilleboe HE. Fat in the diet and mortality from heart disease; a methodologic note. N Y State J Med. 1957;57:2343–2354.

120. DiNicolantonio JJ. The cardiometabolic consequences of replacing saturated fats with carbohydrates or Ω-6 polyunsaturated fats: Do the dietary guidelines have it wrong? Open Heart. 2014 Feb 8;1(1).

121. Mandini S, Conconi F, Mori E, Myers J, Grazzi G, Mazzoni G. Walking and hypertension: greater reductions in subjects with higher baseline systolic blood pressure following six months of guided walking. PeerJ. 2018;6(5):e547.

122. Meerman, R., Brown, A.J., When somebody loses weight where does the fat go? BMJ 2014; 349:g7257

123. Fung, J. (2016) The Obesity Code; unlocking the secrets of weight loss.

124. Osterberg KL, Melby CL. Effect of acute resistance exercise on post-exercise oxygen consumption and resting metabolic rate in young women [published correction appears in Int J Sport Nutr Exerc Metab 2000 Sep;10(3):360]. Int J Sport Nutr Exerc Metab. 2000;10(1):71-81.

125. Melanson EL, MacLean PS, Hill JO. Exercise improves fat metabolism in muscle but does not increase 24-h fat oxidation. Exerc Sport Sci Rev. 2009;37(2):93-101.

126. Ge Long, Sadeghirad Behnam, Ball Geoff D C, da Costa Bruno R, Hitchcock Christine L, Svendrovski Anton et al. Comparison of dietary macronutrient patterns of 14 popular named dietary programmes for weight and cardiovascular risk factor reduction in adults: systematic review and network meta-analysis of randomised trials BMJ. 2020; 369:m696

127. Shapiro, A, Mu., W., Roncal, C., et al Fructose induced Leptin resistance induces obesity in high subsequent fat diets; Am J Comp Physiol 2008 Nov:295(5):1370-5

128. Thau L, Sharma S. Physiology, Cortisol. [Updated 2020 Mar 24]. In: StatPearls [Internet]. Treasure Island (FL): StatPearls Publishing; 2020 Jan-.

129. Heilbronn LK, Smith SR, Martin CK, Anton SD, Ravussin E. Alternate-day fasting in nonobese subjects: effects on body weight, body composition, and energy metabolism. Am J Clin Nutr. 2005;81(1):69-73.

130. Hartman M, Veldius J, Johnson M, augmented Growth homone secretion, frequency and Amplitude mediate enganced GH secretion during a two day fast in normal men. J of Clin Endand Metab. 1992. 74;(4) 757-765.

131. Johnson JB, Summer W, Cutler RG, et al. Alternate day calorie restriction improves clinical findings and reduces markers of oxidative stress and

inflammation in overweight adults with moderate asthma [published correction appears in Free Radic Biol Med. 2007 Nov 1;43(9):1348. Tellejohan, Richard [corrected to Telljohann, Richard]]. Free Radic Biol Med. 2007;42(5):665-674.

132. Ames BN, Cathcart R, Schwiers E, et al. Uric acid provides an antioxidant defense in humans against oxidant- and radical-caused aging and cancer: a hypothesis. Proc Natl Acad Sci USA.1981;78(11):6858-6862.

133. Lloyd-Mostyn R, Lord P, Glover R. Uruca acid metabolism in starvation. Ann. Rheum. Dis. 1970; 29; 553

134. Murray, D. The strange Death of Europe. 2017. Bloomsbury press.

135. Wooden, J. and Jamison S. Wooden; A lifetime of observations and reflections on and ff the court. McGraw Hill. 1997.

136. Buettner D, Skemp S. Blue Zones: Lessons From the World's Longest Lived. Am J Lifestyle Med. 2016;10(5):318–321.

137. Passarino G, De Rango F, Montesanto A. Human longevity: Genetics or Lifestyle? It takes two to tango. Immun Ageing. 2016;13:12.

138. Steves CJ, Spector TD, Jackson SH. Ageing, genes, environment and epigenetics: what twin studies tell us now, and in the future. Age Ageing. 2012;41(5):581–586.

139. Willcox BJ, Willcox DC, Todoriki H, et al. Caloric restriction, the traditiona Okinawan diet, and healthy aging: the diet of the world's longest-lived people and its potential impact on morbidity and life span. Ann N Y Acad Sci. 2007;1114:434–455.

140. Tuberoso CI, Boban M, Bifulco E, Budimir D, Pirisi FM. Antioxidant capacity and vasodilatory properties of Mediterranean food: the case of Cannonau wine, myrtle berries liqueur and strawberry-tree honey. Food Chem. 2013;140(4):686–691.

141. Chiva-Blanch G, Arranz S, Lamuela-Raventos RM, Estruch R. Effects of wine, alcohol and polyphenols on cardiovascular disease risk factors: evidences from human studies. Alcohol Alcohol. 2013;48(3):270–277.

142. www.bluezones.com.

143. Pew Research Center, April 2, 2015, "The Future of World Religions: Population Growth Projections, 2010-2050" .

144. Bruce MA, Martins D, Duru K, Beech BM, Sims M, Harawa N, et al. (2017

Church attendance, allostatic load and mortality in middle aged adults. PLoS ONE 12(5): e0177618.

145. Li S, Stampfer MJ, Williams DR, VanderWeele TJ. Association of Religious Service Attendance With Mortality Among Women. JAMA Intern Med. 2016;176(6):777–785.

146. Wen W, Schlundt D, Andersen SW, Blot WJ, Zheng W. Does religious involvement affect mortality in low-income Americans? A prospective cohort study. BMJ Open. 2019;9(7):e028200.

147. Hill TD, Ellison CG, Burdette AM, Taylor J, Friedman KL. Dimensions of religious involvement and leukocyte telomere length. Soc Sci Med. 2016;163:168-175.

148. Freedman A, Nicolle J. Social isolation and loneliness: the new geriatric giants: Approach for primary care. Can Fam Physician. 2020;66(3):176-182.

149. Holt-Lunstad J, Smith T, Baker M et al. (2015). Loneliness and Social Isolation as Risk Factors for Mortality: A Meta-Analytic Review. Perspectives on Psychological Science, 10(2), 227–237.

150. ec.europa.eu/jrc/en/research/crosscutting-activities/fairness

151. Patel SS, Clark-Ginsberg A. Incorporating issues of Elderly Loneliness into the COVID-19 Public Health Response. Disaster Med Public Health Prep. 2020;1-3.

152. McEwen BS. Central effects of stress hormones in health and disease: Understanding the protective and damaging effects of stress and stress mediators. Eur J Pharmacol. 2008;583(2-3):174–185.

153. Hirotsu C, Tufik S, Andersen ML. Interactions between sleep, stress, and metabolism: From physiological to pathological conditions. Sleep Sci. 2015;8(3):143-152.

154. Epel ES, Blackburn EH, Lin J, et al. Accelerated telomere shortening in response to life stress. Proc Natl Acad Sci USA. 2004;101(49):17312-17315.

155. Greene G. 2004. A Burnt-Out Case. Vintage.

156. Jonsdottir IH, Sjörs Dahlman A. Mechanisms in Endocrinology: Endocrine and immunological aspects of burnout: a narrative review. Eur J Endocrinol. 2019;180(3):R147–R158.

157. Salvagioni DAJ, Melanda FN, Mesas AE, González AD, Gabani FL, Andrade SM. Physical, psychological and occupational consequences

of job burnout: A systematic review of prospective studies. PLoS One. 2017;12(10):e0185781.

158. Shanafelt TD, Hasan O, Dyrbye LN, et al. Changes in Burnout and Satisfaction with Work-Life Balance in Physicians and the General US Working Population Between 2011 and 2014 [published correction appears in Mayo Clin Proc. 2016 Feb;91(2):276]. Mayo Clin Proc. 2015;90(12):1600-1613.

159. Partch CL, Green CB, Takahashi JS. Molecular architecture of the mammalian circadian clock. Trends Cell Biol. 2014;24(2):90–99.

160. Fiona E. Belbin, Gavin J. Hall, Amelia B. Jackson, Florence E. Schanschieff, George Archibald, Carl Formstone, Antony N. Dodd. Plant circadian rhythms regulate the effectiveness of a glyphosate-based herbicide. Nature Communications, 2019;10(1) .

161. Jonathan M Philpott, Rajesh Narasimamurthy, Clarisse G Ricci, Alfred M Freeberg, Sabrina R Hunt, Lauren E Yee, Rebecca S Pelofsky, Sarvind Tripathi, David M Virshup, Carrie L Partch. Casein kinase 1 dynamics underlie substrate selectivity and the PER2 circadian phosphoswitch. eLife, 2020;9.

162. Cappuccio FP, D'Elia L, Strazzullo P, Miller MA. Sleep duration and all-cause mortality: a systematic review and meta-analysis of prospective studies. Sleep. 2010;33(5):585–592.

163. Wennberg AMV, Wu MN, Rosenberg PB, Spira AP. Sleep Disturbance, Cognitive Decline, and Dementia: A Review. Semin Neurol. 2017;37(4):395–406.

164. Ferrie JE, Shipley MJ, Cappuccio FP, et al. A prospective study of change in sleep duration: associations with mortality in the Whitehall II cohort. Sleep 2007;30:1659-66.

165. Emens JS, Eastman CI. Diagnosis and Treatment of Non-24-h Sleep-Wake Disorder in the Blind. Drugs. 2017;77(6):637–650.

166. National Academies of Sciences, Engineering, and Medicine; Health and Medicine Division; Board on Population Health and Public Health Practice; Committee on Public Health Approaches to Reduce Vision Impairment and Promote Eye Health; Welp A, Woodbury RB, McCoy MA, et al., editors. Making Eye Health a Population Health Imperative: Vision for Tomorrow. Washington (DC): National Academies Press (US); 2016 Sep 15. 3, The Impact of Vision Loss. Available from: https://www.ncbi.nlm.nih.gov/books/

REFERENCES

NBK402367/

167. Mullington JM, Simpson NS, Meier-Ewert HK, Haack M. Sleep loss and inflammation. Best Pract Res Clin Endocrinol Metab. 2010;24(5):775–784.

168. Poteser M, Moshammer H. Daylight Saving Time Transitions: Impact on Total Mortality. Int J Environ Res Public Health. 2020;17(5):1611.

169. Walker M. 2017. Why we Sleep. Penguin.

170. Kripke DF, Garfinkel L, Wingard DL, Klauber MR, Marler MR. Mortality associated with sleep duration and insomnia. Arch Gen Psychiatry 2002;59:131-6.

171. Bliwise DL, Young TB. The parable of parabola: what the U-shaped curve can and cannot tell us about sleep. Sleep. 2007 Dec;30(12):1614-5.

172. Naska A, Oikonomou E, Trichopoulou A et al. Siesta in Healthy Adults and Coronary Mortality in the General Population. Arch Intern Med. 2007;167(3):296–301.

173. Leng Y, Wainwright NW, Cappuccio FP, et al. Daytime napping and the risk of all-cause and cause-specific mortality: a 13-year follow-up of a British population. Am J Epidemiol. 2014;179(9):1115–1124.

174. Yetish G, Kaplan H, Gurven M, et al. Natural sleep and its seasonal variations in three pre-industrial societies. Curr Biol. 2015;25(21):2862–2868.

175. Harvey AG, Tang NK. (Mis)perception of sleep in insomnia: a puzzle and a resolution. Psychol Bull. 2012;138(1):77–101.

176. Victorelli S, Passos JF. Telomeres and Cell Senescence - Size Matters Not. EBioMedicine. 2017;21:14–20.

177. Van Deursen JM. The role of senescent cells in ageing. Nature. 2014;509(7501):439–446.

178. Winterbourn CC, Kettle AJ, Hampton MB. Reactive Oxygen Species and Neutrophil Function. Annu Rev Biochem. 2016;85:765-792.

179. Rahal A, Kumar A, Singh V, et al. Oxidative stress, prooxidants, and antioxidants: the interplay. Biomed Res Int. 2014;2014:761264.

180. Broer L, Codd V, Nyholt DR, et al. Meta-analysis of telomere length in 19,713 subjects reveals high heritability, stronger maternal inheritance and a paternal age effect. Eur J Hum Genet. 2013;21(10):1163-1168.

181. Lapham K, Kvale MN, Lin J, et al. Automated Assay of Telomere Length Measurement and Informatics for 100,000 Subjects in the Genetic Epidemiology Research on Adult Health and Aging (GERA) Cohort. Genetics. 2015;200(4):1061–1072.

182. Turner KJ, Vasu V, Griffin DK. Telomere Biology and Human Phenotype. Cells. 2019;8(1):73.

183. Srinivas N, Rachakonda S, Kumar R. Telomeres and Telomere Length: A General Overview. Cancers (Basel). 2020;12(3):558.

184. Babizhayev MA, Savel'yeva EL, Moskvina SN, Yegorov YE. Telomere length is a biomarker of cumulative oxidative stress, biologic age, and an independent predictor of survival and therapeutic treatment requirement associated with smoking behavior. Am J Ther. 2011;18(6):e209-e226.

185. Rode L, Nordestgaard BG, Bojesen SE. Peripheral blood leukocyte telomere length and mortality among 64,637 individuals from the general population. J Natl Cancer Inst. 2015;107(6).

186. Cawthon RM, Smith KR, O'Brien E, Sivatchenko A, Kerber RA. Association between telomere length in blood and mortality in people aged 60 years or older. Lancet. 2003;361(9355):393-395.

187. Rehkopf DH, Dow WH, Rosero-Bixby L, Lin J, Epel ES, Blackburn EH. Longer leukocyte telomere length in Costa Rica's Nicoya Peninsula: a population-based study. Exp Gerontol. 2013;48(11):1266–1273.

188. Lee J, Sandford AJ, Connett JE, Yan J, Mui T, Li Y, et al. (2012) The Relationship between Telomere Length and Mortality in Chronic Obstructive Pulmonary Disease (COPD). PLoS ONE 7(4): e35567.

189. Shammas MA. Telomeres, lifestyle, cancer, and aging. Curr Opin Clin Nutr Metab Care. 2011;14(1):28–34.

190. Werner CM, Hecksteden A, Morsch A, et al. Differential effects of endurance, interval, and resistance training on telomerase activity and telomere length in a randomized, controlled study. Eur Heart J. 2019;40(1):34–46.

191. Honka MJ, Bucci M, Andersson J, et al. Resistance training enhances insulin suppression of endogenous glucose production in elderly women. J Appl Physiol (1985). 2016;120(6):633–639.

192. Leung CW, Laraia BA, Needham BL, et al. Soda and cell aging: association between sugar-sweetened beverage consumption and leukocyte telomere

length in healthy adults from the National Health and Nutrition Examination Surveys. Am J Public Health. 2014;104(12):2425-2431.

193. Cassidy A, De Vivo I, Liu Y, et al. Associations between diet, lifestyle factors, and telomere length in women. Am J Clin Nutr. 2010;91(5):1273-1280.

194. Lee JY, Jun NR, Yoon D, Shin C, Baik I. Association between dietary patterns in the remote past and telomere length. Eur J Clin Nutr. 2015;69(9):1048–1052.

195. Farzaneh-Far R, Lin J, Epel ES, Harris WS, Blackburn EH, Whooley MA. Association of marine omega-3 fatty acid levels with telomeric aging in patients with coronary heart disease. JAMA. 2010;303(3):250-257.

196. Mundstock E, Sarria EE, Zatti H, et al. Effect of obesity on telomere length: Systematic review and meta-analysis. Obesity (Silver Spring). 2015;23(11):2165–2174.

197. Rode L, Nordestgaard BG, Weischer M, Bojesen SE. Increased body mass index, elevated C-reactive protein, and short telomere length. J Clin Endocrinol Metab. 2014;99(9):E1671–E1675.

198. Müezzinler A, Zaineddin AK, Brenner H. Body mass index and leukocyte telomere length in adults: a systematic review and meta-analysis. Obes Rev. 2014;15(3):192–201.

199. Valdes AM, Andrew T, Gardner JP, et al. Obesity, cigarette smoking, and telomere length in women. Lancet. 2005;366(9486):662–664.

200. Denis GV, Hamilton JA. Healthy obese persons: how can they be identified and do metabolic profiles stratify risk?. Curr Opin Endocrinol Diabetes Obes. 2013;20(5):369-376.

201. Furukawa S, Fujita T, Shimabukuro M, et al. Increased oxidative stress in obesity and its impact on metabolic syndrome. J Clin Invest. 2004;114(12):1752-1761.

202. Matsuzawa Y, Shimomura I, Nakamura T, Keno Y, Kotani K, Tokunaga K. Pathophysiology and pathogenesis of visceral fat obesity. Obes Res. 1995;3 Suppl 2:187S-194S.

203. Matsuzawa Y. Pathophysiology and molecular mechanisms of visceral fat syndrome: the Japanese experience. Diabetes Metab Rev. 1997;13(1):3-13.

204. Hoshi A, Inaba Y. Nihon Eiseigaku Zasshi. 1995;50(3):730-736.

205. Miller MA, Croft LB, Belanger AR, et al. Prevalence of metabolic syndrome in retired National Football League players. Am J Cardiol. 2008;101(9):1281-1284.

206. Clemente, D.B.P., Maitre, L., Bustamante, M. et al. Obesity is associated with shorter telomeres in 8 year-old children. Sci Rep 9, 18739 (2019).

207. Mason AE, Hecht FM, Daubenmier JJ, et al. Weight Loss Maintenance and Cellular Aging in the Supporting Health Through Nutrition and Exercise Study. Psychosom Med. 2018;80(7):609-619.

208. Laimer M, Melmer A, Lamina C, et al. Telomere length increase after weight loss induced by bariatric surgery: results from a 10 year prospective study. Int J Obes (Lond). 2016;40(5):773-778.

209. Galkin F, Mamoshina P, Aliper A, de Magalhães JP, Gladyshev VN, Zhavoronkov A. Biohorology and biomarkers of aging: current state-of-the-art, challenges and opportunities Ageing Res Rev. 2020;101050.

210. Ray KS, Singhania PR. Glycemic and insulinemic responses to carbohydrate rich whole foods. J Food Sci Technol. 2014;51(2):347–352.

211. Ditzen B, Hoppmann C, Klumb P. Positive couple interactions and daily cortisol: on the stress-protecting role of intimacy. Psychosom Med. 2008;70(8):883-889.

212. Hertenstein MJ, Keltner D, App B, Bulleit BA, Jaskolka AR. Touch communicates distinct emotions. Emotion. 2006;6(3):528-533.

213. Floyd K. Relational and Health Correlates of Affection Deprivation. Western Journal of Communication. 2014 Jul;78(4):383-403.

214. Field T, Diego M, Hernandez-Reif M. Preterm infant massage therapy research: a review. Infant Behav Dev. 2010;33(2):115-124.

215. Hansen GM, Egeberg A, Holmstrup P, Hansen PR. Relation of Periodontitis to Risk of Cardiovascular and All-Cause Mortality (from a Danish Nationwide Cohort Study). Am J Cardiol. 2016;118(4):489-493.

216. Loos BG, Van Dyke TE. The role of inflammation and genetics in periodontal disease. Periodontol 2000. 2020;83(1):26-39.

217. Chang Y, Lee JS, Lee KJ, Woo HG, Song TJ. Improved oral hygiene is associated with decreased risk of new-onset diabetes: a nationwide population-based cohort study. Diabetologia. 2020;63(5):924-933.

218. Li C, Lv Z, Shi Z, et al. Periodontal therapy for the management of

cardiovascular disease in patients with chronic periodontitis. Cochrane Database Syst Rev. 2017;11(11):CD009197.

219. McRaven W. Make your Bed. 2017. Penguin.

ADDITIONAL READING

1. Blackburn E and Epele. 2017. The Telomere Effect. Orion Spring.

2. Buettner D. 2012. The Blue Zones, Second Edition: 9 Power Lesson For Living Longer From The People Who've Lived The Longest. National Geographic.

3. Carey N. 2012. The Epigenetics Revolution. Icon Books.

4. Karnazes D. 2006. Confessions of An All-Night Runner. Penguin.

5. Davis W. 2011. Wheat Belly. Rodale.

6. Duhigg C. 2012. The Power of Habit. Random House Books.

7. Fitzgerald M. 2014. Run Stronger and Faster By Training Slower. 80/20 Running. New American Library; Penguin.

8. Fung J and Noakes. 2016. The Obesity Code: Unlocking the Secrets of Weight Loss.

9. Goldacre B. 2009. Bad Science. Harper Perennial.

10. Greene G. 2004. A Burnt-Out Case. Vintage.

11. Havil J. The Irrationals: A Story of the Numbers you can't count. Princeton University Press. 2012.

12. House S, Johnston S, Jornet. 2019. Training for The Uphill Runner. Patagonia Works.

13. Hitchens C. 2008. God Is Not Great. Atlantic Books.

14. Hodgkinson T. 2005. How to Be Idle. Penguin.

15. Lustig R. 2013. Fat Chance. Hudson Street Press.

16. Plomin R. 2018. Blueprint: How DNA Makes Us What We Are. Penguin.

17. McRaven W. 2017. Make Your Bed. Penguin.

18. Mischel W. 2014. The Marshmallow Test. Penguin.

19. Murray D. The Madness of Crowds. 2019. Bloomsbury Publishing.

20. Murray D. The Strange Death of Europe. 2017. Bloomsbury Publishing.

21. Peterson J. 2018. 12 Rules for life: an antidote for chaos. Random House.

22. Spector T. 2015. The Diet Myth. Weidenfeld & Nicolson.

23. Walker M. 2017. Why We Sleep. Penguin.

24. Wallman J. 2015. Stuffocation. Penguin.

25. Wooden J and Jamison S. 1997. A lifetime of Observations and Reflections On and Off the Court Hardcover. McGraw Hill.

INDEX

Printed in Great Britain
by Amazon

45522063R00203